Praise for *The Peanut Allergy Answer Book*

"Parents of children with peanut allergy, as well as individuals with food allergy themselves, will find this book an invaluable resource. The question-and-answer format reflects interactions which often occur at a doctor's visit and the questions included are those which repeatedly occur in discussions regarding peanut allergy. The format provides a ready resource to be referred to in a casual, un-rushed fashion, and one which will be used repeatedly by individuals faced with peanut allergy."

"Publications regarding food allergy are sometimes vague and may be misleading. Dr. Young has provided, in a straightforward and scientifically documented way, accurate and timely information regarding not only peanut allergy but also a wide range of food allergy questions. Food allergy and anaphylaxis are often emotionally charged and anxiety-provoking problems which will be easier to face with a reference such as this available."

FRANK J. TWAROG, M.D., PH.D.
Associate Clinical Professor, Harvard Medical School
Senior Associate in Medicine (Immunology), Children's Hospital, Boston

"It was a pleasure to read *The Peanut Allergy Answer Book*. It is a collection of illustrative cases of peanut anaphylaxis that should be read by every parent with a child suffering from this affliction....It is the most thoughtful, readable review currently available of this intrusive, occasionally fatal allergic disorder."

ALBERT SHEFFER, M.D.
Clinical Professor of Medicine, Harvard Medical School
Allergy and Clinical Immunology, Brigham and Women's Hospital, Boston

"*The Peanut Allergy Answer Book* is an excellent resource for patients and families. It provides practical easy-to-understand answers and advice for common peanut allergy questions. The case examples highlight the common scenarios encountered by peanut-allergic patients. This book presents up-to-date scientifically-based information which will be helpful to anyone who wants to learn more about peanut allergy."

LYNDA C. SCHNEIDER, M.D.
Director, Allergy/Clinical Immunology Program, Children's Hospital, Boston
Assistant Professor of Pediatrics, Harvard Medical School

"Peanut allergy has been increasing in prevalence during the past few decades. Due to the potential severity of peanut-induced allergic reactions and its wide use in many unlabeled foods, patients often accidentally ingest peanuts. This heightens the anxiety of everyone involved.... Until now, there has been no single resource explaining all aspects of peanut allergy. This cutting-edge book

i

provides the answers to the many questions that patients, their parents and other interested people have in the management of peanut allergy....Whether read in its entirety or selectively for answers to specific questions, I encourage anyone interested in peanut allergy to use this book as a resource for better understanding of this condition."

DONALD Y. M. LEUNG, M.D., PH.D.
Head, Division of Pediatric Allergy-Immunology,
National Jewish Medical and Research Center
Professor of Pediatrics, University of Colorado Health Sciences Center
Editor-in-Chief, The Journal of Allergy and Clinical Immunology

"A wonderful little book, chock full of important and up-to-date information that should be read not only by the peanut allergic patient, but by all patients with food allergy. Food allergy patients will find this book not only education-al, but helpful in the diagnosis and treatment of their disease. Although a valu-able tool for all food allergy sufferers, this book should also be read by all healthcare providers who are involved with treating food allergy patients. I will certainly recommend this book to my patients and colleagues."

JAMES P. ROSEN, M.D.
Assistant Clinical Professor of Pediatrics,
University of Connecticut Medical School

"Dr. Michael C. Young, a premier allergy physician in New England, has put together an outstanding book that provides the essential information for patients with peanut allergy. This includes not only the latest scientific infor-mation, but also practical information about how to deal with problematic issues, from airline travel and school lunches to emergency treatment. All of this is presented in a format that is accurate, concise, and readily understand-able. I am certain that my patients with peanut allergy will find a wealth of tips and useful advice in this book. *The Peanut Allergy Answer Book* is required reading for all patients with peanut allergy and their parents!"

DALE T. UMETSU, M.D., PH.D.
Professor of Pediatrics
Chief, Division of Allergy and Clinical Immunology
Director, Center for Asthma and Allergic Diseases,
Stanford University

THE PEANUT ALLERGY
ANSWER BOOK

THE
PEANUT ALLERGY
ANSWER BOOK

MICHAEL C. YOUNG, M.D.

FAIR WINDS
PRESS

GLOUCESTER, MASSACHUSETTS

First published in the USA in 2001 by
Fair Winds Press
33 Commercial Street
Gloucester, Massachusetts 01930

Library of Congress Cataloging-in-Publication data available
British Library Cataloging-in-Publication data available

First Edition

10 9 8 7 6 5 4 3 2 1

Printed and bound in the United States

ISBN 1-931412-58-8

*This book is not intended to replace the services of a physician.
Any application of the recommendations set forth in the following pages
is at the reader's discretion. The reader should consult with his or her own
physician or specialist concerning the recommendations in this book.*

TABLE OF CONTENTS

CHAPTER 3

ANAPHYLAXIS

CHAPTER 4

FINDING THE HIDDEN PEANUT
PRODUCTS

CHAPTER 5

KEEPING SAFE IN A PEANUT-FILLED
WORLD

CHAPTER 6

PREVENTION OF PEANUT AND OTHER FOOD ALLERGIES

CHAPTER 7

THE FUTURE OF PEANUT ALLERGY

DEDICATION

This book is dedicated to my loving wife and daughter
and to my father, who have provided me with their
encouragement, inspiration, and love.

I also dedicate this book to the loving memory of my mother,
who gave up her career as a young physician to raise
my sister and me, and inspired us to the call
of medicine and learning.

ACKNOWLEDGMENTS

One of the true pleasures of practicing the specialty of allergy is having patients who are genuinely interested in finding out the causes and triggers of their problems rather than just treatments and cures. Allergy patients are especially interested in learning about their problems and how to prevent them. Over the years, I have had the privilege of caring for many patients and their families. I have learned much from all of them and they are directly responsible for this book. I would like to extend my deepest gratitude to all of my patients.

In particular, I would like to thank Christopher Smith, a peanut-allergic toddler and his mother, Lisa Lavieri, who looked for a book on peanut allergy and was unable to find one. She discussed this with her sister, Holly Schmidt, a publisher of health books, who then contacted me to write this book. I owe Christopher, his mom, and his Aunt Holly a special thanks.

I gratefully acknowledge and thank all my teachers and colleagues, especially my mentors during my allergy fellowship training at Boston Children's Hospital: Drs. Raif Geha; Donald Leung; Frank Twarog; and Martin Broff; who gave me the opportunity to join his practice.

I also thank my colleagues for reviewing this book and giving helpful comments and suggestions: Drs. Martin D. Broff, Raif S. Geha, Donald Leung, Frank Twarog, James Rosen, John S. Saryan, Lynda Schneider, Albert L. Sheffer, S. Allan Bock, Hugh Sampson, and Dale Umetsu.

I have a special word of thanks to Anne Muñoz-Furlong. As the founder of the Food Allergy Network, she is the model of what a dedicated parent can do. She has single-handedly revolutionized the field of food allergy by forming the most important organization in the field which serves patients, the medical community, and the general public. For her achievements, Anne was awarded the Distinguished Layperson Award in 2000 by the American Academy of Allergy, Asthma and Immunology. I am privileged not only to have had Anne review this book and assist me with her many helpful and thoughtful comments, but to have her write the foreword as well. If my patients provided me with purpose in writing this book, Anne gave me inspiration. I gratefully acknowledge her contributions not only to this book but to all people with food allergies. I also thank Michele Carrick, who as the mother of a severely allergic son with peanut anaphylaxis and asthma, became very active in the Allergy and Asthma Foundation of America, and who kindly reviewed this book and gave many useful comments.

I thank Holly Schmidt, my publisher at Fair Winds Press, who not only gave me the opportunity to write this book, but with her patient teaching, greatly improved my writing and helped shape this book in its early stages of development.

I acknowledge my dedicated nursing and office staff, and my associates, Drs. Martin D. Broff, Catherine O'Brien and Jon E. Stahlman for their support and friendship.

Finally, I thank my family, especially my wife Karen and my daughter Liane, whose understanding and love provide me with the inspiration for all that I do.

FOREWORD

Much has been written in the press about food allergy, specifically peanut allergy, in the past five years. Too often, however, the stories focus on controversial issues or miracle cures. Often they leave the reader with many unanswered questions. *The Peanut Allergy Answer Book* will change that.

This book, written for patients; parents; and lay people who are interested in peanut allergy, is based on scientific data and reports cutting–edge research. It clearly and simply explains many of the questions you may have been asking yourself, including: "What is peanut allergy?," "Is it increasing?," "Did I cause my child's peanut allergy?," "Will there be a cure?," and more. Dr. Young has done a thorough review of research studies and presents the findings throughout the book in an easy-to-understand format.

The Peanut Allergy Answer Book will be a wonderful resource for anyone who is interested in learning more about peanut allergy. Whether you are newly diagnosed or have been living with this allergy for a lifetime, it's bound to be a book you will refer to over and over again.

Anne Muñoz-Furlong
Founder, *The Food Allergy Network*

INTRODUCTION

The number of peanut-allergic people I treat as an allergist has dramatically increased in the past few years. Where I might have routinely seen one or two patients a month with peanut allergy just five years ago, I now often see more than one or two patients a week. I sometimes see one or two a day for the same problem. Most of the people with peanut allergy I saw ten or more years ago were adults. Now my peanut-allergic patients, particularly those with new peanut allergies, are exclusively very young children and infants. The number of people, especially young children, with life-threatening allergic reactions has also dramatically increased. There has been heightened interest in peanut allergy, especially with the recent attention focused on banning peanuts from schools and airlines. There are a number of explanations for the increasing numbers of peanut-allergic people. One of these is the very high consumption of peanuts and peanut products all over the world. More than five billion pounds of peanuts are produced each year in the United States alone which is more than any other country. According to the United States Peanut Council, eleven pounds of peanut products are ingested annually by the average American. About fifty-five percent of peanuts are consumed in the form of peanut butter and the remainder are consumed as table nuts, in baked goods, and in sweets. Peanuts and peanut products, especially peanut butter, are an inexpensive and convenient food source and have become very popular as snacks and quick meals, often substituting for regular full meals in many busy households. Infants and young children become exposed to peanut products, especially peanut butter, very early in life. As a result of this increased exposure to peanuts and peanut products, particularly peanut butter, the number of people allergic to peanuts has greatly increased in the past ten years. Peanut allergy is unfortunately a potentially life-threatening allergy and for most children, a lifelong problem that is usually not outgrown.

When Holly Schmidt, my publisher at Fair Winds Press, first approached me to write this book, I was surprised to learn that there were no available books specifically on the subject of peanut allergy. From the large numbers of patients I follow in my private practice in Massachusetts and in the Allergy Program at Boston Children's Hospital, I knew there was a definite need for a comprehensive book on this subject. This book is written for the increasing number of people with peanut allergies and their families. It addresses the many issues they face, from knowing what foods contain peanut and peanut products; to understanding how to deal with peanut exposures in daycare, schools, and airlines; to performing emergency planning in the event of a life-threatening allergic attack. In my practice and in my reading of the medical and consumer literature, I found people asking the same questions. This book is written and organized in a question-and-answer format to address those commonly-asked questions. I have tried to make medical terms easy to understand.... Use the glossary in the back of the book for new terms. Many of these new words are bold-faced in the text. From reading this book, you will learn how to successfully prevent and manage this problem and thus will not have to live in constant fear of life-threatening exposures. You will learn all you need to know about peanuts and allergies and will be able to design strategies to cope with this allergy. I have my many patients to thank for the inspiration for these questions and for the concept of this book.

CHAPTER 1

ALLERGIES IN A NUTSHELL

WHAT IS FOOD ALLERGY?

Matthew is a six-month-old baby who has been breast-fed since birth. At two months of age, his mother introduced rice cereal into his diet with no problems. Subsequently, she gave him oatmeal and applesauce, and at five months of age he had egg for the first time. He developed a very itchy dry scaly rash on his face which, over the course of several weeks, worsened to involve the creases of his arms, the backs of the knees and his neck and ears. His pediatrician diagnosed "baby eczema" and pre-scribed a moisturizer and hydrocortisone cream. The rash improved but did not resolve. It seemed to worsen with food, but there was no consistent pattern. His mother brought him to my office and allergy tests showed he was allergic to milk, soy, egg white, wheat, and peanut. His rash significantly improved with the elimination of these foods from his diet.

The symptoms of food allergy in children typically involve the skin. Hives are common, particularly on areas of contact such as the mouth, lips, and face. In severe cases, these areas can become swollen and intensely itchy. When the skin becomes chronically inflamed, the rashes take the form of eczema, a very itchy dry, scaly eruption that often begins in early infancy. Typical areas of skin involvement are the face; arms and legs, particularly the creases; knees and elbows; neck; and behind the ears. Gastrointestinal symptoms are also common, ranging from nausea, vomiting and diarrhea to acute abdominal pain and colic. More subtle reactions can take the form of failure to eat and gain weight. Respiratory symptoms, such as wheezing, nasal congestion, and mucous secretion, are less common chronically but can be severe when they occur acutely. Some people with asthma have food allergy and their asthma can be triggered by the ingestion of the foods to which they are sensitized. Conversely, some people with food allergy who do not have asthma can experience an asthma-like reaction when they eat the foods they are allergic to. When these people are studied, they often have an asthmatic tendency, although their baseline lung function will usually be normal. This means that, although they do not have the diagnosis of asthma, they may be prone to chest symptoms such as chronic cough or wheezing with common colds, physical activity and exercise. Finally, anaphylaxis, or a life-threatening systemic allergic reaction can occur. It is rare, but is, of course, the most dangerous of all allergic reactions and what we all work to prevent and avoid.

Food allergy is more common in children than in adults. It has been estimated that six to eight percent of infants younger than age two are allergic to food, and approximately 1.5 percent of adults have food allergy. The common food allergens in children are milk, eggs, soy, wheat, and peanut. Of these, milk, eggs, and peanuts cause eighgty percent of all food allergies in children. In adults, the common food allergens are tree nuts, peanut, fish and shellfish, which cause eighty-five percent of allergic reactions. A recent survey in the United States suggests that 0.7 percent of children are allergic to peanuts. Sensitivity to many foods, especially milk, eggs, and soy tend to resolve with age, whereas allergy to peanuts and tree nuts often begins in infancy but fails to improve with age. For reasons that are still unclear, peanut allergy is associated with fatal anaphylaxis more than any other food.

Food allergies usually occur in individuals who also have other manifestations of allergic disease such as hay fever, asthma, and eczema. People with these allergic disorders have a greater tendency to develop sensitivities to food. Since allergies tend to be inherited, family members are often allergic as well although not necessarily with the same allergies. Although allergies to specific foods are not inherited per se, the tendency to be allergic to food in general is genetic. Some recent studies now suggest the possibility of genetic transmission of peanut allergy, but results are still inconclusive.

WHAT IS FOOD ALLERGY AND HOW DOES IT RELATE TO THE IMMUNE SYSTEM?

Richard is a 43-year-old man who had milk allergy as a child and was affected by eczema and chronic diarrhea. On a milk-and-dairy-free diet, he eventually outgrew these symptoms and was able to consume milk products by the time he entered school. He had no further allergy problems until he developed hay fever and asthma at age thirteen. These symptoms remain unchanged and are usually worse in the spring when the trees pollinate. He also has hives and wheezing when he is near cats and dogs. He has a two-year-old son with chronic eczema and recurrent ear infections, who recently developed hives from peanut butter.

People commonly think of allergies as sneezing, itchy watery eyes, and stuffy noses that occur when they get "hay fever" in the spring and fall. Some other people wheeze and have trouble breathing from asthma attacks when they exercise or when they "feel allergic." Still others become deathly ill when they are stung by bees and yellow jackets. How do all these different problems relate to the person who is unable to eat certain foods, such as peanuts or shellfish, because they break out in hives, experience swelling of their throat, or have abdominal pain and diarrhea?

These reactions are all results of the body's immune system reacting in an inappropriate way to what should be innocent and innocuous things in our daily lives. That is what an allergy is. In order to understand how this happens, we need to learn a little bit about how our immune system works and how this can cause us to get allergies to different things. We will learn the definition of a few key words such as allergen, IgE, mast cells, and histamine.

The immune system is responsible for protecting the human body from infection and invasion from bacteria, viruses, and other harmful agents by its ability to distinguish "self" from "nonself." Substances identified as foreign or "nonself" are attacked by cells of the immune system and destroyed or rendered inactive. The immune system in allergic people is different from that of nonallergic individuals in that innocuous and benign things, such as food, pollen, animal dander, and medications, are identified as harmful to the body and targeted for an immune response. This response is a very potent inflammatory reaction that results from the production of a special protein called **IgE** which recognizes a specific allergic agent (**allergen**) in the same way that antibodies recognize bacteria and viruses. This recognition is very specific because a given IgE protein is unique to one and only one allergen. So, peanut-specific IgE will recognize only peanut, and cat-specific IgE will recognize only cat. This is the reason why some people are allergic to certain things but not to others. What things a person is allergic to are determined by what specific types of IgE proteins he has; so that someone allergic to peanuts will react to peanuts only and not to cat unless he also has cat-specific IgE. This IgE protein circulates in our bloodstream throughout our whole body and finds its way to various tissues and organs such as the skin, gastrointestinal tract, lungs, nose, and eyes. On reaching these areas, the IgE attaches to cells called **mast cells** which are located in these organs and tissues. Once the allergen-specific IgE is attached to the mast cells, a person becomes "sensitized" to that particular allergen.

Mast cells are important in allergies because they make the chemical **histamine** as well as other **mediators**. Histamine and other mediators are what directly cause the many symptoms of allergies such as itching, hives, stuffy nose, and wheezing. We use **antihistamines** because they are medications that block the actions of histamine, thereby blocking allergic symptoms. When the sensitized tissues come in contact with the allergen—through eating or breathing for example—the allergen attaches to the tissues by means of the allergen-specific IgE mast cell complex. This attachment causes the mast cell to release large amounts of histamine and other similar chemical mediators into the blood. Histamine circulates through the blood and to surrounding tissues and subsequently binds to these tissues by means of histamine receptors. Antihistamines work by inhibiting the binding of histamine to these tissue receptors.

Histamine binding results in many tissue reactions and changes. In the nose and eyes, congestion, swelling, mucous secretion, itching and sneezing result. In the lungs: constriction of air passages results in shortness of breath, wheezing, and difficulty breathing. In the gastrointestinal tract: vomiting, diarrhea, and abdominal cramping result. In the skin: itching, swelling, hives, and eczema result.

In the most severe reaction, the cardiovascular system is affected with a drop in blood pressure, shock, and potentially death. This potentially fatal reaction is called **anaphylaxis**. The allergens that are the most common causes of life-threatening anaphylaxis are the allergens that are absorbed into the body internally such as food, medications, insect stings and, in certain instances, latex rubber. Of the foods, the most potent allergens are peanuts, tree nuts, seafood, and shellfish. These are the foods most commonly associated with anaphylaxis and, of these, peanut is number one on the list. The treatment and prevention of anaphylaxis will be discussed in later chapters.

HOW DO YOU KNOW IF YOU
HAVE A FOOD ALLERGY?

I have always loved all kinds of seafood especially shellfish. I was attending a meeting of allergists and had just returned to my hotel room following a delicious buffet luncheon where quite a bit of seafood had been served and where, following my appetite, I had indulged myself, especially in the lobster and crab dishes. I noticed that my entire chest and abdomen were suddenly intensely itchy and hot. I noted on my watch that approximately 30 minutes had gone by since I had finished lunch. I took off my shirt and was surprised to see myself covered with large red hives. I looked in the mirror and saw that my entire body was bright red. At this time, I also felt my heart racing and a tightness in my throat. "This must be what early anaphylaxis must feel like!" I thought. I had never felt this way before. Luckily, I had some antihistamine samples I had gotten earlier in the meeting. I took two tablets and tried not to panic. After all, I was at an allergy meeting full of allergists! Surely, someone must have epinephrine! Fortunately, the itching and hives started to recede and, after a long hour, I felt much better but quite sleepy from the side effects of the antihistamine. I missed the rest of the meeting that day. The following morning, my allergist colleagues asked me where I was. Apparently, I had missed an interesting lecture on food allergies! Later that week, when I returned to work, I skin-tested myself with our panel of common allergenic foods. I had a positive skin test to crabmeat only and was negative to everything else. In the six years since that incident, I have meticulously avoided crabmeat but have eaten all other shellfish and seafood with no problems. I recently repeated the skin test to crabmeat and it was negative. However, I have not attempted to eat crabmeat yet.

Food allergies are usually recognized initially by the person or his family. Allergic symptoms such as itching; rashes such as hives or eczema; abdominal pain; nausea; vomiting; diarrhea; and breathing difficulty are all common symptoms of food allergy. When the symptoms occur in a consistent and recognizable pattern, following the ingestion of a specific food, it then becomes obvious that food allergy may be the cause of the various symptoms the person is experiencing. For example, ingestion of peanuts can result in the immediate eruption of hives, swelling, and difficulty breathing. This is not subtle and you can make the diagnosis easily. When the symptoms are chronic and inconsistent, it may be less clear whether or not the cause is due to a specific individual food or several foods, or perhaps not even to food at all. Seeing an allergy specialist to assist in the diagnosis or to document suspected food allergy may be very helpful. The allergist can sort through confusing symptoms and make deductions and conclusions on the basis of your history. He can also perform allergy testing to confirm the presence of specific food allergies. The allergy specialist has the special training to do this.

HOW DO I CHOOSE AN ALLERGIST?

An allergist specializes in the diagnosis and treatment of allergic diseases and asthma. Allergists complete an additional six years of specialty training after receiving their medical degree. An allergist needs to complete allergy specialty training and pass the board examinations in either internal medicine or pediatrics before being allowed to take the allergy board examination. Allergy specialty training consists of two to three additional years of training in allergy and immunology in fellowship programs. During this time, the doctor will learn about how to diagnose and treat hay fever, asthma, eczema, food, drug, and insect allergies in children and adults. Choosing a board-certified allergist will ensure that the doctor has completed the required allergy and immunology training and passed the examination for the allergy specialty. Your primary care physician is the best person to contact regarding a referral to the best local allergist for you. Your primary care physician would have an established relationship with that doctor and know his or her particular style and expertise with allergy patients. Your doctor may know the allergy specialist's particular interests which may include food allergies. The American Academy of Allergy, Asthma, and Immunology (www.AAAAI.org) and the American College of Allergy, Asthma, and Immunology (www.ACAAI.org) are national organizations of allergy specialists and they can give you names of all the allergists in your local area. Other organizations that can be helpful with referrals to allergists are the Allergy and Asthma Foundation of America and the American Lung Association as well as your local medical society.

As with selecting any adviser, whether a doctor, lawyer, accountant, or broker, you want to meet the allergist first and talk to him or her to determine whether there is compatibility, compassion, and trust. A good doctor will *listen* to you above all and allow you to speak freely about your problem and all your concerns regarding it. The art of good medicine is to be able to take a good history from the patient, and you can tell a lot about the doctor's knowledge from his or her questions. Frequently, good questions can help guide you to think about the problem better and, ultimately, you might be able to come up with answers yourself. If you are a parent, observe the doctor's ability to relate to the child and whether or not a rapport develops. Never underestimate the ability of a child to describe his or her observations. A good doctor experienced with children can elicit this history effectively even from small children. Go to the doctor's appointment with a specific list of questions and concerns. Write things down! Things always seem more confused and hectic during the appointment so having something concrete to refer to will make things much smoother and easier.

WHAT INFORMATION DOES YOUR DOCTOR NEED TO DIAGNOSE FOOD ALLERGY?

Doctor, I have food allergies!
Please describe your symptoms.
I have nausea and pain in my stomach every time I eat.
Have you noticed which foods cause these symptoms?
I can't really tell, it seems that all meals will do it.
How soon after you eat do you feel the nausea and stomach pain?
Sometimes it's during the meal and other times, it's a few hours afterwards.
Do you have any other symptoms along with the nausea and pain such as itching, hives, swelling, or difficulty breathing or swallowing?
Yes, but I get those all the time, not just with eating!

Food allergy symptoms can be very difficult to sort through, and often the symptoms are very vague and nonspecific in nature, making it difficult for you and your doctor to diagnose. The key to solving this puzzle is a history carefully taken by an allergist or a physician with experience in dealing with food allergies. The physician will take a detailed history of your symptoms, paying special attention to the sequence of reactions and correlating the timing of your symptoms with the specific foods eaten. Severely allergic people usually experience their reactions within 30 to 60 minutes after they eat. Delayed symptoms sometimes occur and this makes it harder to determine which food is the cause of the reaction. In this situation, it is the consistency and pattern of responses that can help clarify what is going on.

ALLERGY TESTS

The suspicion of food allergy can be verified by performing allergy tests on the person. Allergy testing is usually performed by an allergy specialist. The allergist has specialized training and certification in the treatment of allergic and immunologic diseases, including the diagnosis and management of food allergies. Documentation of specific food allergies can be done by either **skin prick tests** and/or IgE **RAST** tests by blood sampling.

The Food Diary

✦ One of the most useful tools in the diagnosis of food allergy, for both the doctor and the patient, is a carefully kept journal in which you record your exact symptoms (itching, hives, nausea, abdominal pain, trouble breathing, etc.), the timing of the first symptoms in relation to meals and eating, and, most importantly, a complete list of everything eaten. Ideally, this should include not only all food and drink items, but also the ingredient lists of processed foods. The reason for this is that, as we'll learn later in this book, there are many "hidden foods and ingredients" contained in products that are not always obvious. Artificial flavoring, dyes, and preservatives can also cause allergic reactions in some people. Recording how much of the food you eat is important, especially the smallest amount that will cause a reaction. The most recent reaction as well as the number of times that a reaction has occurred with each food is also helpful. Review of this information can give great insight into whether or not specific foods are responsible for specific symptoms. Often, hidden sources of exposure, such as cross-contamination, can be deduced from a carefully recorded food diary. Food diaries can also be helpful in assessing chronic conditions, such as eczema or chronic gastroenteritis, in which acute exacerbations and attacks may be rare.

In skin testing, a very dilute extract of the actual food is used. The allergenic extract material is processed and purified by commercial laboratories. A drop of the liquid extract is placed on the skin and a plastic or metal point is then used to prick the skin just enough for the extract material to penetrate the skin without actually breaking the skin. If the person is allergic to the extract material, his or her skin mast cells will already be sensitized to it and the person will have a histamine-mediated reaction. The histamine will cause a small hive where the skin was pricked in the skin test.

When performing skin tests, your allergist will also administer a positive control with histamine to demonstrate that the skin is capable of reacting. The normal skin response of all people is to have a reaction to histamine with some itching and redness and a small hive. In some situations, however, the skin response to histamine is blocked or diminished and the skin will not respond to any allergen testing either. The most common situation in which the histamine response is absent occurs when you have taken antihistamine medication before the skin tests. You should stop antihistamine medications five to seven days prior to skin tests; otherwise, your histamine response, as well as your response to any potential allergen tests, will be blocked. You doctor will also administer a negative control with saline (a salt water solution) to control for the possibility of false positive skin tests caused by certain sensitive skin conditions. Skin tests can be read in twenty minutes, are inexpensive, and minimally uncomfortable with minor itching being the main effect. In children younger than two years, the skin may not always be reactive and false negative skin tests may result. Some doctors suggest that in the case of a negative skin test, the skin test should be repeated using a fresh sample of the actual food as there may be loss of activity or potency in the manufacturing process of the extract material.

IgE RAST Tests

Blood tests used to diagnose allergies are referred to as the RAST test which stands for " radioallergosorbent test." The original technique involved radioactive reagents, but most laboratories currently use non-radioactive "tracers" that rely on color changes in the reagents. The test works by detecting the presence of allergen-specific IgE in the blood. Blood is drawn from the arm and sent to the laboratory where it is processed. This involves adding the blood to the allergen which has been attached to a paper dish, plastic plate, or cellulose matrix. Following a timed interval, this mixture is washed and a "tracer" anti-IgE antibody is added to detect the binding of your IgE to the allergen. The amount of allergen-specific IgE contained in the blood sample can be calculated from this result. How high, or positive, the RAST test is reflects how much antibody the patient has to that specific allergen. Although the RAST test is more expensive and less accurate than skin prick tests, they can be useful in people who are unable to stop antihistamine therapy, people who have extensive skin disease or people in whom there is a significant risk of anaphylaxis from the skin testing. The main problem with RAST tests is that the results can vary considerably from laboratory to laboratory because of differences in laboratory technique and procedure as well as in quality control. A modified type of RAST test, called the CAP RAST system, has recently been shown to more accurately measure the degree and severity of allergy to four foods: peanut, milk, egg, and fish. Best of all, it correlates with the results of double-blind placebo-controlled food challenges which are explained later. For the four foods studied, there is preliminary evidence to suggest that the levels of allergen-specific IgE measured by the CAP system may correlate with how active your symptoms are and if these levels decline, it may indicate that you are losing the allergy. CAP RASTs may ultimately be a better way of following food allergies since skin tests can remain positive even when clinical activity lessens as a child "outgrows" the food allergy.

The Best Test

The definitive method of diagnosing food allergy is the **double-blind placebo-controlled food challenge (DBPCFC)**. It is useful to understand the DBPCFC method because it is referred to frequently in the food allergy literature. The DBPCFC is a functional test that seeks to reproduce the patient's actual symptoms by direct challenge. Therefore, it can be useful in the diagnosis of non-IgE mediated food reactions such as lactose intolerance as well as classical food allergies. The DBPCFC method eliminates the possibility of patient bias and investigator bias by "blinding" both sides so that neither the patient nor the investigator knows whether the actual food or a placebo (a dummy sample that contains no food protein) is being given. There are many symptoms and reactions that can be mistaken for food-allergic reactions so it is important to be able to objectively assess and separate these reactions from true allergic reactions.

To illustrate this concept, Dr. K. Rix and his colleagues in Great Britain studied twenty-three patients with a history of food reactions. All patients were able to consistently identify the foods that triggered their reactions. However, when the foods were administered blindly through a tube directly into the stomach, the only four individuals who had any symptoms were the four who had convincing histories of anaphylaxis. Five of the nineteen nonresponders walked out of the study when it became obvious they were not reproducing their allergic symptoms with the food they claimed to be allergic to.

The placebo effect is another important factor that can complicate any medical study. A **placebo** is the so-called "sugar pill" or "dummy pill" that contains no active ingredient, whether it be medication or food substance. Its purpose in a challenge test or medical study is to measure the person's response to what he or she *believes* to be the real food or medication. Placebos can cause many different symptoms such as cough, headache, itching, wheezing, and high blood pressure. There are studies showing that people can be addicted to placebos. The placebo effect has been shown to be thirty-five percent, which is higher than many medicines on the market! Therefore, any scientifically sound study has to account for the placebo effect by using a control group of patients who are given placebo in a "blinded" fashion so they do not know whether they are being given the study food or a placebo. The food or placebo is given in a capsule that is tasteless, giving no clue to its contents. For young children, the food is hidden in a carrier such as applesauce. The code telling what each capsule contains is sealed until the end of the study. The challenges are usually done with escalating doses. Once the study with both food and placebo capsules is completed, the seal on the code is broken and the results can be tabulated. If the person's symptoms are reproduced with the food and not with the placebo, using the DBPCFC method, the diagnosis of the food-specific allergy can be made.

The danger of any challenge method is the possibility of inducing anaphylaxis in the allergic individual. Obviously, challenges should be done only in a medical facility capable of treating anaphylaxis. If the actual amount of food that caused the reaction is known, graded smaller concentrations of the food can be used sequentially in the challenge procedure, building up to the actual amount that was originally ingested. This increases the safety of the procedure. From a scientific point of view, the DBPCFC is considered the "gold standard" for the diagnosis of food allergy. Although the DBPCFC can be performed in your allergist's office, it is usually performed in a hospital setting.

WHAT IS AN ELIMINATION DIET?

Andrew is three-years-old and has had severe eczema since the age of six months. He was evaluated in my office last month and skin tests showed allergies to milk and eggs. I recommended eliminating all milk and egg products from his diet. On his follow-up appointment, he still had significant eczema, although it was less extensive than before his diet change. On close questioning, it appeared that he was still eating some baked goods at his grandmother's that were cooked with milk and eggs. Once this was eliminated, Andrew's eczema was much easier to control.

When you suspect food allergies, but are not entirely certain which foods are the cause, an elimination diet can be the answer. An elimination diet completely and strictly eliminates each suspect food for a certain time period. You should make the original list of suspect foods from a careful analysis of your food and symptom diary and your medical history. If the symptoms persist despite a carefully done elimination diet, screening allergy tests such as skin prick tests or IgE RAST tests might help narrow down the list or screen for foods that were not originally suspected. Once you make a list of suspect foods, you and your physician can design an elimination diet. The diet has to be completely free from the suspect foods, including products containing and cooked with the foods, and all possible hidden sources of the foods. The greater the number of foods eliminated, the more difficult the elimination. Ideally, the challenge period should be two weeks. If your symptoms resolve during that period of elimination, you have found a possible cause. If the symptoms persist despite the elimination diet, it is unlikely that the suspect foods were relevant and you might then proceed to other possible foods. An elimination diet should only be done under a physician's supervision to avoid the possibility of any nutritional deficiencies.

Elemental Diets

If the elimination diet to select foods was unsuccessful in resolving the symptoms, the next step would be going on an elemental diet. Elemental diets are essentially allergen-free formulas that are nutritionally complete in proteins, fats, and carbohydrates. Examples of elemental infant formulas are Neocate® and Elecare®. Pregestimil®, Alimentum®, and Nutramigen® are hypoallergenic formulas that do contain small protein fragments or peptides. For adults, Vivonex® is available as well. An elemental diet is a rather extreme alternative but if it fails to resolve your symptoms, you can be reasonably sure you don't have a food allergy.

If the symptoms do resolve, the next step is to reproduce the symptoms by direct challenge. This is ideally done by DBPCFC but an open challenge can be considered if the skin or RAST test is negative and the actual history is rather doubtful for allergy. In this situation, the risk for anaphylaxis is low and the challenge is fairly safe to perform in the office. Food challenges should never be done at home if there is even a remote chance of anaphylaxis or severe symptoms occurring.

The confirmed diagnosis of a food allergy is made when the elimination of the offending food resolves the symptoms and when challenge with the offending food reproduces the symptoms.

ARE THERE FOOD REACTIONS THAT AREN'T ALLERGIES?

It is important to remember that reactions to foods can occur by mechanisms other than allergic reactions. Food intolerance can occur in individuals whose digestive system is unable to digest and metabolize food, resulting in undigested or partially digested food which can then lead to bacterial overgrowth, diarrhea, gas formation, and abdominal pain and cramping. Lactose intolerance is probably the most common example of this, occurring in five percent of the Caucasian population but in as much as sixty to ninety percent of Blacks, Hispanics, and Asians. Since people with lactose intolerance are unable to digest lactose, the major sugar in milk, they often mistakenly believe that their intolerance of milk is actually a milk allergy. Although milk avoidance is the treatment plan for patients with lactose intolerance just as it is for milk-allergic patients, the mechanisms for their respective problems are very different. Since skin testing and RAST testing will only detect allergen-specific IgE, these tests will not be helpful in the diagnosis of food intolerances and other types of adverse food reactions in which IgE is not involved. Skin tests and RAST tests performed on these individuals will be negative. Most children with milk allergy will outgrow the problem. Most people with lactose intolerance have it as a permanent condition. Many, however, are able to tolerate varying amounts of dairy products in their diets depending on the severity of their particular condition.

CHAPTER 2

PEANUT ALLERGY 101

WHAT IS THE HISTORICAL BACKGROUND OF PEANUT ALLERGY?

Peanuts were cultivated for food at least as early as 2,000 to 3,000 B.C. The American biochemist George Washington Carver (1860–1943) is given credit for developing the many modern uses of peanuts. He was interested in enriching the nutrition of minorities and the poor, and peanuts provide a highly nutritious and inexpensive source of easily digestible protein. Peanuts are also an excellent source of vitamin B-12 (niacin), vitamin E, magnesium, chromium, and manganese. These nutrients are typically found in meats, whole grains, legumes, and vegetable oils. The peanut's versatility and ability to be prepared in so many forms—eaten whole as a vegetable; roasted and salted as a snack; crushed and ground as a spread or "butter," and incorporated into candy, baked goods and other foods—was ideal for Dr. Carver. It could also be used for cooking oil which was extracted by pressure or solvents. Dr. Carver discovered more than 300 uses for the peanut, including the manufacturing of plastics, adhesives, bleaches, and linoleum among others. In addition, the cultivation of peanuts and the manufacturing of peanut products were important sources of employment and remain so to the present. The United States, particularly the southern states, remains one of the world's largest producers of peanuts.

The History of Peanut Allergy
in Medicine

As early as the fourth century B.C., Hippocrates observed that milk could induce hives and gastric upset. Food allergy was described as a clinical entity in 1921 by Prausnitz and Kustner. The first definite reference to nut allergy in medical literature was in 1920 by the noted hematologist Dr. Kenneth Blackfan. He observed a ten-year-old child with eczema that was "always intensified" by nuts, eggs, and fish. "The eating of any of them was followed almost immediately by a burning sensation in the throat, vomiting, diarrhoea, oedema of the lips and ears, and urticaria." There was no research in the field of peanut allergy until as recently as 1976 when May performed food challenges on asthmatic children and showed that peanut-allergic patients developed asthma symptoms when challenged with peanuts. In 1978, Bock reported fourteen children with peanut allergy proven by direct challenge. In 1981, Taylor reported ten patients with peanut allergy who ingested encapsulated peanut oil without any allergic reactions, suggesting that peanut oil was not allergenic. In 1984, Sampson and Albergo showed that positive skin prick tests and RAST tests to peanut correlate 100 percent with positive challenge to peanut, establishing the usefulness of these allergy tests in the diagnosis of peanut allergy. In 1988, Yunginger reported fatal anaphylaxis to food in seven patients, four of whom turned out to have peanut allergy. In 1992, Sampson reported thirteen patients with food allergies, five of whom had peanut allergy. Of the six patients with fatal anaphylaxis, three were allergic to peanuts. Both reports emphasized the great risk in delaying the administration of epinephrine to patients experiencing anaphylaxis. In 1989, Bock and Atkins showed that peanut allergy in childhood usually persists into adulthood. In 1992, Leung and his colleagues reported three patients with peanut anaphylaxis successfully treated with immunotherapy to peanut extract. However, the rate of systemic reactions to the therapy was very high at thirteen percent. More recent work has focused on the immunology and molecular biology of peanut allergy, characterizing the specific proteins causing IgE-mediated reactions. This research has led to successful gene sequencing and cloning of peanut protein. Using this information, several laboratories are working on potential vaccines for peanut allergy and other potential techniques for treatment, and biotechnology laboratories in the food industry are working on a nonallergenic peanut. If you are interested in learning more about the studies mentioned in this chapter or throughout the rest of the book, please see Appendix D.

HOW COMMON IS PEANUT ALLERGY?

Current estimates show that approximately 0.5 percent to 0.7 percent of children in the United States and the United Kingdom and up to two to five-million Americans are affected by peanut allergy. Sicherer's 1999 telephone survey study showed a 1.1 percent prevalence of peanut and nut allergy in the United States, or approximately three million Americans, including both children and adults. The prevalence of peanut allergy alone is 0.6 percent of the population. A British study showed that one in 200 four-year-olds have peanut allergy. One percent of all British preschool students are estimated to be affected. Infants and toddlers are particularly susceptible to peanut allergy. A recent study showed that peanut-allergic patients had their first allergic reaction at an average age of twenty-two months. A study of eighty-one children with a history of food allergies by May and Bock showed that twenty-one percent of these patients had peanut allergy by double-blind food challenges. In adults, a recent national survey in the United States by Sampson showed that 1.3 percent of adults are allergic to peanuts and tree nuts. Comparing peanut allergy to other food allergies, 2.5 percent of newborn infants are allergic to cow's milk in the first year of life, and 15 percent retain this allergy into their second decade of life. Egg allergy occurs in 1.3 percent of children. Shellfish allergy occurs in approximately 0.5 percent of the population. Peanuts are by far the most common cause of food anaphylaxis.

Frequency of Food Allergies in Children:

Milk	2.5%
Egg	1.3%
Peanut	0.6%
Shellfish	0.5%

Another study found that of 185 infants, eighty percent had been exposed to peanut products by age one year and 100 percent had exposure by age two years. Follow-up at age seven showed that seven percent of high-risk children tested positive to peanut, and four percent had definite reactions to peanut by history or actual challenge. Dr. Hugh Sampson, a prominent investigator in the field of food allergy and director of The Jaffe Food Allergy Institute at New York's Mount Sinai School of Medicine, has observed an increase of fifty-five percent in the number of peanut-allergic children over the past ten years, and the number of allergic reactions to peanuts in both children and adults has increased by ninety-five percent over the same time span. This increased prevalence of peanut allergy is consistent with the reports of allergists across the country as well as worldwide.

IS PEANUT ALLERGY HEREDITARY?

Peter is a 31-year-old man with a lifelong history of peanut and tree nut allergy. His mother and sister have food allergies but not to peanut. His wife has hay fever but no food allergies. She is pregnant with their first child, and they would like to know what their baby's chances of developing peanut allergy are.

It is well-known that allergic diseases, such as asthma; hay fever; and eczema, cluster in families, and the individual often inherits one or more of the allergic diseases together. Food allergy is inherited, but whether allergies to specific foods, such as peanut, are inherited has not been extensively studied. Dr. Jonathan O'B. Hourihane, a prominent British peanut allergy researcher from the University of Southampton, examined fifty peanut-allergic children and their forty-nine mothers, forty-eight fathers and forty-five siblings with questionnaires and skin prick tests. This study showed that all types of allergic diseases become more common in successive generations and occur more often in your maternal relatives than your paternal relatives. You are more likely to suffer from peanut allergy if one of your siblings has it than if one of your parents is allergic. The study showed that not only is peanut allergy inherited but also the tendency for all the other allergic diseases as well. Most recently, a report by Dr. Scott Sicherer and his colleagues at Mount Sinai School of Medicine in New York examined seventy-four identical and fraternal twin pairs with peanut allergy recruited from the Food Allergy Network. Among identical twins, both twins were peanut allergic in sixty-four percent of cases whereas in fraternal twins, the concordance rate was seven percent, which is the same as the concordance rate of nontwin siblings. These results strongly indicate the significant genetic influence on peanut allergy. Although I am not routinely recommending that all symptom-free siblings of a peanut-allergic child be tested for peanut allergy, I feel it is reasonable if the family requests it for their own reassurance. More studies have to be performed before a general policy on testing siblings is universally accepted.

HOW EARLY CAN PEANUT SENSITIZATION OCCUR?

Caitlin's mother first suspected Caitlin was allergic to peanuts when each time after eating peanut or peanut butter herself and then breast-feeding Caitlin, the baby became very irritable, and when Caitlin was four-weeks-old, she developed an itchy red rash on her face, which also flared up after breast-feeding. At that point, her mother stopped eating peanut products. Caitlin was weaned completely from breast milk by six months of age. She was kept away from all peanut products until she was two-years-old. The very first time she was given peanut butter on a cracker, she developed hives all over her body and had some wheezing as well. She was referred to me by the emergency room physician who treated her for that reaction.

Sensitization to peanut can occur very early in life. One theory is that this may be due to the high potency of the peanut allergens. One study showed that eighty percent of peanut-allergic individuals developed allergic symptoms on their first known exposure. A French study of newborn infants younger than eleven days and babies between age seventeen days and four months showed that eight percent had positive skin tests to peanut. This certainly implies that sensitization occurred either shortly after birth or in the womb. One very interesting study by Hourihane from the United Kingdom showed a correlation between the self-reported increased consumption of peanuts by pregnant and nursing mothers and a definite decrease in the age of onset of peanut allergy over the last ten years. In other words, the more peanut products consumed by pregnant and nursing mothers, the younger the age at which their children developed their peanut allergies. Studies show that the fetus is capable of being sensitized to milk protein. Although the studies on peanut have not yet been done, peanut protein is such a potent allergen that it is more than likely capable of doing the same. Therefore, a pregnant mother's diet can affect her child's likelihood of developing food allergies.

Eating Peanuts While Breast-feeding

Peanut proteins can be detected in breast milk for several hours after the mother has eaten peanuts. What this means is that an exclusively breast-fed baby can still be exposed to peanut protein and become sensitized to peanut through the mother. Babies with peanut allergies can develop allergic symptoms following nursing if the mother has recently eaten peanuts. Since a family history of allergic disorders, such as hay fever, asthma, and eczema, is a risk factor for the development of food allergy, it may be prudent for the pregnant and nursing woman with this type of family history to avoid allergenic foods such as peanut. For more information information on breast-feeding, see page 85.

Other potential routes of sensitization are peanut-oil-based vitamin preparations and infant formula. These items are a problem primarily in Europe and are mentioned here to alert the traveler who might unknowingly make purchases of products that normally would not contain peanut oil in the United States. A report from France studied 122 children ages seven months to five years old. During the first two years of life, one group of children received vitamin D free from peanut oil, and two groups received vitamin D containing peanut oil. The two groups receiving vitamin D containing peanut oil had positive skin tests to peanut while the group receiving peanut-oil-free vitamin D had significantly less sensitization on skin testing. Most American brands of vitamins, such as Flintstones Supplements®, One-A-Day®, and Bugs Bunny Vitamins® do not contain peanut oil. There is a report on the presence of allergenic peanut oil in milk formula in the British medical journal *Lancet* from 1991, but, to my knowledge, no American infant formulas contain peanut oil. It is important to always be cautious when traveling abroad because of different practices in foreign countries. Topical creams and lotions can also contain peanut oils. Children with damaged skin due to chronic inflammatory skin conditions, such as eczema, are probably most susceptible to sensitization from topical preparations. Most pharmaceutical-grade peanut oils contain no detectable levels of peanut protein but it is certainly possible that the low levels of peanut protein that can cause sensitization are too low to be detectable by available technology.

WHAT IN PEANUTS MAKE THEM SO ALLERGENIC?

John is a 25-year-old man with a lifelong history of peanut and tree nut allergies as well as egg, wheat, and soy allergies. He had an anaphylactic reaction at age thirteen when he was accidentally given some brownies that had nuts in them. He has been extremely careful about avoiding all nuts since then without any further problems. He has had mild hives with egg, wheat, and soy products, but never anaphylaxis.

The answer lies in the part of the peanut that actually causes the allergy—he peanut proteins. Allergic reactions result from our body's immune responses to proteins; most food-allergic reactions are triggered by food proteins. In milk, the milk proteins are casein and the major whey proteins are lactalbumin and lactoglobulin. In egg white, they are ovalbumin and ovomucoid. In wheat, it is gluten and in shrimp, it is tropomyosin. The allergenic peanut proteins are the seed storage proteins vicilin, conglutin, and glycinin. By understanding the nature of these peanut proteins, scientists are beginning to unlock the mystery of why peanuts are among the most potent of all food allergens. The protein content of a peanut is 24.3 percent of the average weight of a peanut. The allergenic proteins in peanuts are found in the cotyledon, or embryonic leaf, of the peanut seed plant. These proteins, like other food allergens, are glycoproteins, which are proteins that have sugars as part of their structure. Work from several laboratories has identified three major allergenic proteins from peanuts called Ara h1, Ara h2, and Ara h3. Ara is derived from arachia, the Latin term for peanut. The genes for these allergens have been cloned and sequenced. Ara h1 belongs to the vicilin family of seed storage proteins, Ara h2 belongs to the conglutin family and, the most recently identified peanut allergen, Ara h3 belongs to the glycinin family. Ninety-five percent of peanut-allergic patients react to Ara h1 and Ara h2 while approximately 50 percent of peanut-allergic patients react to Ara h3. Scientists have discovered some structural features of Ara h1 and the way it binds to IgE that explain why it is such an extremely allergenic protein. With this information, researchers are now working on ways to alter the structure of this protein and hope that, in doing so, a "hypoallergenic peanut" might be created that retains all the characteristics of a peanut except for causing allergic reactions. There is also research being conducted on creating vaccines to these peanut allergens.

IS THE PEANUT A TRUE NUT?

Peanuts are vegetables and nuts are fruits. Peanuts (botanical name *Arachia hypogea*) are actually members of the legume family which includes lentils, soybeans, peas, black-eyed peas, chick peas, lima beans, kidney beans, green beans, and garbanzo beans. Peanuts are native to South America and several varieties are grown in the United States. These include the Virginia, Spanish, and runner variety. Peanuts grow in the ground unlike tree nuts which grow on trees. The peanut plant is an bushy, flowering annual. After fertilization, the flower stalk elongates until its weight causes it to bend down touching the ground. Continued growth of the stalk pushes the ovary into the ground and the seeds grow, forming the familiar peanuts.

The botanical definition of a true nut is a hard, dry, closed one-seeded fruit. In general, the term nut can apply to any seed or dried fruit of a woody plant that does not belong to the legume family. The tree nuts commonly eaten are walnuts, almonds, cashews, pecans, Brazil nuts, hazelnuts, and pistachios. Almonds, pecans, and pistachios are the seeds of fruits. The fruit contains a pit that encloses the nut. Almonds come in two types: sweet almond which is the edible kind, and bitter almonds which are poisonous (although the oil can be extracted and is safe to use). Walnuts come in three varieties: black, English, and Persian walnuts. Pecans are related to hickory nuts and are covered by a leathery skin. Brazil nuts are the seed of large woody fruits. They include creamnut; chestnut of Para; and sapucaia, or paradise nut. The cashew nut is the seed of a pearlike fruit that must be roasted to be palatable. The pistachio, sometimes known as the green almond, is also the seed of a drupe like the almond and pecan. Piñon, or pine nuts are the seeds of pines and are found in pine cones. Pignolia nuts are the seeds of the European pine and resemble pine nuts. The hazelnut, or filbert, is a true nut and is the seed of a pearlike green fruit. Other true nuts are acorns, beechnuts which are primarily used for animal feed, and chestnuts. Macadamia nuts are also called Queensland, Australian Gympie, Bush, and Bopple nuts. The seed is contained in a fruit with a fleshy husk, and the thin shell of the seed is cracked to release the nut. The coconut is also the seed of a fruit but is generally not restricted from the diet of tree-nut-allergic people. Nuts found in other parts of the world are ginkgo nuts used in Chinese and Asian cooking; Pili or Javanese almonds; and terminalia, or wingnuts, found in the Orient. Water chestnuts, nutmeg, and mace are not nuts and do not need to be avoided by tree-nut-allergic people. Although many people are allergic to more than one nut, some people have just one solitary tree-nut allergy.

SHOULD ALL MEMBERS OF A FOOD FAMILY BE AVOIDED IF YOU ARE ALLERGIC TO ONE FOOD IN THAT FAMILY?

Anne is thirty-six and recently married a Greek man who brings her to visit his family in Athens every summer. She has developed allergy symptoms to some Greek dishes experiencing hives, diarrhea, and on one occasion, wheezing. She thinks she is allergic to some of the spices such as parsley, dill, caraway, and anise. Her food skin tests were positive to celery and carrots, both members of the Umbelliferae family to which parsley, dill, caraway, anise, coriander, and fennel also belong. She tries to avoid all members of this food family, but has trouble convincing her Greek mother-in-law of her allergy problem.

The prevailing thought at one time was that being allergic to one type of legume meant that you would cross-react to all members of the legume family regardless of previous exposure or history. Since peanuts are legumes, people allergic to peanuts were therefore advised to avoid not only peanuts but all members of the legume family whether or not they had ever had a reaction to other legumes. To take this logic further, it was also a common belief that being allergic to one member of a food group automatically made you allergic to every food in that group. This theory was based on the work by Vaughan and Black in 1929 when they classified foods into botanically related food groups. They concluded that cross-reactions would occur between foods belonging to the same food family similar to the cross-reactions observed in pollen allergies.

Recent studies by Bock and others at the National Jewish Medical and Research Center in Denver, Colorado, show that this type of cross-reactivity does not commonly occur. Sampson of the Jaffe Food Allergy Institute in New York studied sixty-nine patients with one or more positive skin tests to legumes and gave them oral double-blind placebo-controlled food challenges in the hospital with five legumes: peanut, soybean, pea, green bean, and lima bean. Only two patients had a positive food challenge to more than one legume. They concluded that clinically relevant cross-reactivity to legumes is very rare and that clinical sensitivity to one legume does not warrant dietary elimination of the entire legume food family unless sensitivity to each food is confirmed by blind oral challenges.

There is one special consideration regarding other legumes. A recent report by Moneret-Vautrin from France demonstrated cross-reactivity between peanut and another legume, the lupines. The lupine is consumed either in the form of seeds or as flour used to supplement wheat flour. Apparently, in France, up to ten percent lupine flour can be added to wheat flour and is not subject to labeling. Lupine flour is used in baked goods, pasta, sauces, milk, and soy substitutes. There have been several reports of lupine allergy. This study examined twenty-four peanut-allergic individuals for lupine allergy and found positive skin prick tests in forty-four percent. In six people challenged by DBPCFC, five were positive to lupine. The blood from four individuals demonstrated RAST inhibition to lupine by peanut, demonstrating cross-reactivity. The authors warn that cross-reactivity to this legume hidden in wheat flour can be a serious problem for the peanut-allergic individual. Read labels of imported foods, especially baked goods, for lupine or lupine flour and avoid them.

You can be allergic to multiple foods, including foods in the same family, but this is usually a result of separate allergies and not a common cross-reacting allergy. In general, you need avoid only the specific food you are allergic to by history, and it is not necessary to avoid the entire food family. The two main exceptions to this recommendation would be the tree nuts and the crustacean shellfish (shrimp, lobster, crab). There does seem to be cross-reactivity among members of these food groups.

Thirty-five percent of peanut-allergic people are also allergic to tree nuts, but only ten percent of peanut-allergic people are allergic to legumes. The rate of cross-reactivity between a tree nut with other tree nuts is greater than fifty percent. Soybeans react with other legumes less than five percent of the time. The rate of cross-reactivity of wheat with other grains is twenty-five percent. Within the animal proteins, beef and lamb cross-react fifty percent of the time, and fish species cross-react with other fish species more than fifty percent of the time.

If you are allergic to peanuts, you should also avoid tree nuts unless allergy testing is negative or unless you have previously tolerated tree nuts. Legumes, however, should be safe to eat even if you have peanut allergy. If you are allergic to one tree nut, avoid all other tree nuts.

ARE PEANUT-ALLERGIC INDIVIDUALS ALSO ALLERGIC TO TREE NUTS?

Investigators studying peanut-allergic individuals have found coexisting tree nut allergies in thirty-four percent to fifty percent of those people, depending on the study. Among patients with tree-nut allergy, twenty-two percent reported having reactions to more than one tree nut. It is unknown whether the coexistence of peanut and tree-nut allergies is due to cross-reacting proteins or whether this reflects a general increase in the tendency to react to highly allergenic proteins in an allergic individual. This may not necessarily be due to specific allergens, such as peanuts or tree nuts, but may apply to all allergenic foods. This is supported by Sampson's study which showed that, of the peanut-and tree-nut allergic population, fifty-seven percent are also allergic to egg, thirty-seven percent are also allergic to milk and twenty-nine percent are also to fish and shellfish. People who are allergic to one food seem to have the tendency to be allergic to others. On the other hand, there is some evidence of cross-reactivity between peanuts, walnuts and pecans.

SHOULD PEANUT-ALLERGIC INDIVIDUALS AVOID TREE NUTS?

Clearly, there are many people with peanut allergy who can eat tree nuts with no problem and many people with tree-nut allergies who can eat peanuts. However, many allergists, myself included, recommend that children allergic to peanuts avoid all tree nuts except for previously tolerated tree nuts or unless testing for those tree nuts is negative. When your peanut-allergic child reaches age five years, testing for tree nuts can be performed or repeated, and if negative, introducing tree nuts into the diet can be considered. This is admittedly a very cautious approach. The rationale for this recommendation is the difficulty in the identification of specific nuts, particularly in mixtures and in processed food, the significant potential for peanuts contaminating other nuts, and the recognition that tree-nut allergy is also potentially severe and lifelong.

CAN PEANUT ALLERGY BE TRANSFERRED FROM PERSON TO PERSON?

In 1997, a case report was published in the *New England Journal of Medicine* of a liver and kidney transplant recipient who developed a new peanut allergy. His donor organs apparently came from a man who had died from peanut anaphylaxis after eating satay sauce containing peanuts. The recipient had no prior history of peanut or food allergy. Three months after his transplant, the patient developed a skin rash and swelling of his throat after eating peanuts. RAST test to peanuts was positive. Interestingly, a woman received a pancreas and the other kidney from the same peanut-allergic organ donor. She never developed peanut allergy and she had a negative RAST to peanut. She was challenged with peanut and had no reaction. The transfer of peanut allergy to the recipient most likely was the result of the transfer of white blood cells contained in the donor liver called B cells which produce peanut-specific IgE. Similar transfer of peanut allergy with bone marrow transplantation has been reported. Because transplant recipients take drugs to suppress their normal immune response to allow survival of the donated organ, cells of the donor immune system are not destroyed by the recipient. This allows cells of the immune system, such as B cells secreting peanut-specific IgE contained in the bone marrow, to survive, and these transplanted cells will perpetuate the peanut allergy in the transplant recipient. In contrast, B cells and other cells of the immune system capable of causing allergies are not found in the pancreas or kidney so these transplants do not transfer allergies from donor to recipient. Blood transfusions present no risk of transferring allergies because transfusion recipients are not immunosuppressed and any donor B cells would be destroyed by the recipient's immune system. For organ recipients, the allergic B cells might eventually be destroyed as the patient's immunosuppressive drugs are tapered. For bone marrow recipients, the allergic B cells are an intrinsic part of the bone marrow so there would never be any improvement in the transferred allergy.

Organ transplant recipients should be warned of the possibility of their developing allergic reactions if their organ donor has a history of food allergies.

WILL I OUTGROW MY PEANUT ALLERGY?

Jason, age five, had peanut allergy diagnosed at age one when he developed hives from just touching his face with peanut butter. He was never exposed to peanut again and was strictly kept away from all peanut and nut products without any accidents and did well. His family never needed to use their Epipen®. He did not have any other allergy-related problems. Jason was about to enter kindergarten and his mother wanted to know whether he was still allergic to peanuts. Skin tests to peanut and tree nuts were negative. He was challenged with peanut butter in the clinic and had no reaction. He can now eat everything without restrictions.

Most studies seem to indicate that peanut allergy, unlike allergies to milk, soy, egg, and wheat, are stable through time and not outgrown. The first study to address the question of the natural history of food allergy was by Dr. S. Allan Bock of the National Jewish Medical and Research Center in Denver, Colorado in 1982. He studied eighty-seven children with proven food allergies. Fifty-six of the children were older than three years and thirty-one children were younger than three years. Age three was chosen as a dividing point for the two study groups because all children older than age three years, in the experience of the National Jewish Medical and Research Center, had IgE-mediated allergic reactions. The study was conducted with telephone interviews and follow-up DBPCFC. The elapsed time from initial testing to the follow-up interview ranged from several months to seven years. In children older than three years, nineteen percent of previously positive food challenges had turned negative at the time of follow-up. The most common foods to become tolerated with age were milk, egg, and soy. Peanut and tree nuts did not improve significantly. In children less than age three years, forty-four percent of the positive food challenges turned negative. Milk, egg, and soy were again the foods that were tolerated with age. Bock concluded that older children diagnosed with food allergy tended not to outgrow their food allergies in contrast to younger children who were more likely to, especially those with milk and egg allergies. In several other studies, older children and adults have been shown to outgrow or lose their food allergies if they are able to completely eliminate the food allergen from their diet. The exceptions to this are the highly allergenic foods such as peanuts, tree nuts, fish, and shellfish.

To address the specific issue of whether peanut allergy is outgrown, Dr. Bock with Dr. Fred Atkins published in 1989, a follow-up study on thirty-two peanut-allergic children aged two years to fouteen years. These thirty-two patients all had impressive histories of peanut-allergic reactions, positive skin prick tests, and positive DBPCFC. Two to thirteen years after their initial evaluation, patients were contacted by telephone and gave updated information on the status of their peanut avoidance measures, their most recent peanut ingestion (both accidental and intentional), resultant symptoms and treatment required, and any subsequent allergy evaluation testing that had been done. All patients interviewed declined requests for repeat DBPCFC. Eight patients had successfully avoided any peanut ingestion. Seven patients had follow-up skin prick tests to peanut, and all remained positive from two to ten years after initial evaluation. Twenty-four patients out of the thirty-two had accidental ingestions and all ingestions resulted in symptoms ranging from skin reactions (hives, swelling, eczema) to gastrointestinal to nasal and eye symptoms to wheezing, coughing and laryngeal edema. No patient had a drop in blood pressure or anaphylaxis. The conclusion of the study is that peanut allergy is long-lasting and does not appear to improve with time.

In 1998, Dr. Hourihane and his colleagues in the United Kingdom studied 120 children ages two years to ten years. They all had a convincing history of peanut allergy and all underwent open peanut challenge. Twenty-two children were identified who had outgrown peanut allergy and documented with negative challenges. Fifteen of these "resolvers" were matched by age with fifteen "persisters," and features of their history and symptoms were compared as well as skin test and serum IgE results. The age of the first reaction to peanut, serum IgE, severity of reactions, and the number of reactions were similar in both groups. There were no cases of anaphylaxis in this study. The time interval between the last reaction and challenge was longer, but not significantly so, in resolvers than persisters. The resolvers also had negative skin test results or smaller results than persisters. The resolvers tended to have fewer food allergies. Hourihane concluded that some preschool children with mild to moderate allergic reactions to peanuts have a 22/120, or eighteen percent, chance of resolving or outgrowing the allergy. Follow-up of fourteen resolvers showed no reactions to peanuts on further peanut exposure. This study is consistent with my own clinical experience and that of others which has shown that young children age two to three years, who become allergic to peanuts only, with mild, nonanaphylactic symptoms, can outgrow their peanut allergy. In my practice, I have found the numbers to be small, on the order of ten percent to twenty percent, comparable to Hourihane's study. The children who become successful resolvers also had meticulous peanut and peanut product avoidance with no accidental ingestions. Sampson has recommended that children who had an isolated peanut reaction in the first two years of life, and who have successfully avoided any further peanut reactions for three years or more, be retested by the CAP RAST and, if the result is low, have skin prick testing done. Depending on the initial reaction history, a challenge can ultimately be performed to document the resolution or persistence of peanut allergy.

In contrast to the young children, other studies, including Bock's, show that when peanut allergy develops in the older child or adult, it does not resolve with time.

✦ Ten to twenty percent of people outgrow or resolve their peanut allergy. These "resolvers" have meticulous avoidance of peanut with nearly no accidental ingestions, smaller skin test results, and fewer food allergies in total. It is possible that the younger your child is when diagnosed with peanut allergy, the better his chances are of outgrowing it.

CHAPTER 3

ANAPHYLAXIS

WHAT IS ANAPHYLAXIS?

At the party, George made sure to ask whether the sugar cookie he ate contained nuts because he had a severe peanut and tree-nut allergy. The hostess assured him they did not since she baked them herself. As soon as he took a bite of the cookie, George knew something was wrong. He felt his lips, tongue, and throat instantly swell and his entire body became intensely itchy. Within a few minutes, he felt chest pain and tightness and he could not breathe. His face and body were bright red and covered with hives. He had the feeling he was going to die. He was able to reach for his Epipen® and inject himself in the thigh before passing out. Luckily his wife had already called 911 and, by the time the paramedics arrived 15 minutes later, George had regained consciousness and could breathe. He received another dose of epinephrine and was transported to the local hospital where intravenous fluids, antihistamines, steroids, and aerosol asthma medications were given over the next 12 hours. He made a full recovery and was able to be discharged the following morning, completely back to normal. Later, the hostess of the party admitted that she had forgotten she had made the sugar cookies in the same mixing bowl that she had previously used to make cookies that contained nuts.

Anaphylaxis is the systemic manifestation of allergy—when an allergic reaction affects the body as a whole and not just locally. In other words, some patients have hives just in the area of contact with the food allergen, such as the lips and mouth, while other patients erupt in hives over their entire body, regardless of the route of exposure. It is this latter systemic total body reaction that is termed anaphylaxis.

The severity of anaphylaxis can be graded mild, moderate, or severe. The symptoms of mild anaphylaxis are hives, a sensation of fullness of the mouth and throat, swelling of the eyelids and lips, and nasal congestion. Moderate anaphylaxis would be accompanied by the additional symptoms of generalized or rapidly worsening hives and itching, swelling, flushing, wheezing, and vomiting. The potential worse-case scenario is severe anaphylaxis which is a life-threatening reaction. This can cause severe swelling of the tissues of the upper airway, resulting in obstruction of breathing through the throat, blocking airflow in and out of the lungs. When the lower airways of the lungs narrow, shortness of breath, wheezing and asthma can occur, further compromising oxygenation. When the cardiovascular system of the body undergoes anaphylaxis, massive fluid leakage from blood vessels into tissue results in decreased blood pressure and shock. Severe anaphylaxis is explosive in onset, usually occurring within minutes after exposure. Patients often have a "sense of impending doom" in the initial stages of severe anaphylaxis. Seizures can result from lack of oxygen. The combination of obstructed breathing and lack of oxygen with loss of heart function and blood pressure is often fatal.

Grades of Anaphylaxis and Treatment

SEVERITY	SYMPTOMS	TREATMENT
Mild	Skin involvement only	Antihistamines
Moderate	Generalized or rapidly progressive skin improvement, respiratory, gastrointestinal	Epipen®, antihistamines, emergency medical attention
Severe	Cardiovascular, shock, death	Epipen®, antihistamines, steroids, emergency medical attention, intensive care

The common causes of fatal anaphylaxis are bee stings, drug reactions, and food allergy. Annually, there are 300 deaths from penicillin allergy, 100 deaths from food allergy, and fifty deaths from insect-sting anaphylaxis. The majority of food anaphylaxis results from peanuts and tree nuts.

There are other conditions that can mimic the symptoms of anaphylaxis. Chest tightness and difficulty breathing can be a symptom of asthma, heartburn, or anxiety. A heart attack is sometimes very similar to an anaphylactic reaction so prompt medical attention by a physician is crucial so that proper and appropriate treatment can be given.

CAN SEVERE ANAPHYLAXIS BE PREDICTED?

Richard had seen an allergist for asthma when he was a child. He had allergy testing then and recalled being told that he was allergic to cats, dogs, dust, and pollen. He never had any problems with food allergy. Two weeks ago, he collapsed while eating at a Chinese restaurant. He was brought to the nearest hospital emergency room and found to be in shock. Tests showed no evidence of a heart attack. His skin showed no evidence of any insect sting, and his lungs were clear with no asthma. He was on no medications. He fully recovered and was discharged in forty-eight hours. He was referred for allergy testing to rule out food anaphylaxis. Skin tests were positive to peanuts, cashews, and almonds. His wife remembered that, on that evening, they had ordered beef satay with peanut sauce and chicken with cashews.

There is unfortunately no available test to predict who is at risk for a life-threatening allergic reaction, short of doing an actual challenge test. The size of skin tests and the severity of positive RAST tests do not correlate with the risk of anaphylaxis. Anyone who is allergic can potentially undergo an anaphylactic reaction. Peanut reactions are often severe, even on the first exposure. Forty percent of first reactions to peanuts involve wheezing and respiratory distress. There are three factors in your history that increase the risk for a severe anaphylactic reaction: (1) a history of previous anaphylaxis, (2) peanut and tree-nut allergy and (3) a history of asthma. If you have these risk factors, you should be extra careful about following your restriction diet, especially when eating outside your home. If you have asthma, make sure it is under good control and be sure you have your asthma rescue inhaler with you at all times. You should keep at least two Epipens® on your person because of the risk that one may misfire or be defective. In addition, one Epipen® dose lasts only twenty to thirty minutes at the most, so in the case of a severe, prolonged reaction or in the event of a late-phase reaction, a second dose may be needed. All peanut-allergic individuals and their families should be prepared to treat anaphylaxis. Since there is no cure for peanut allergy, strict avoidance is the key to management.

WHAT IS THE TREATMENT FOR ANAPHYLAXIS?

Dennis knew as soon as he bit into the candy that something was wrong. His lips and the inside of his mouth began to itch and burn. His tongue and throat felt swollen within a minute, despite his downing a glass of water. He knew this was serious and he had to get to his car where he kept his Epipen®. Running out the door, he started to wheeze with each breath. He was fumbling for his keys when he felt he was going to pass out. The last thing he remembered was injecting himself in the thigh with the Epipen® as he fell to the pavement.

———————

Clearly, avoidance is the best treatment plan. Documenting the exact allergens responsible for the reactions, and gaining understanding and insight into where the allergens are located (and hidden!) is the key to any successful plan. This is the subject of another chapter which will deal with this crucial matter in detail. Once the allergic exposure has occurred and symptoms follow, certain steps need to be followed to prevent severe, potentially fatal anaphylaxis. In the case of mild anaphylaxis where primary involvement is in the skin, a rapid-acting antihistamine is often all that is necessary. Antihistamines block the binding of histamine to tissue receptors which is what causes the actual symptoms of allergy such as itching, redness, hives, and swelling. Examples of antihistamines available without prescription are diphenhydramine (Benadryl®) and chlorpheniramine (Chlortrimeton®). Benadryl® is commonly used for food-allergic reactions because it is very effective for skin reactions and works rapidly, usually within an hour. It is a very safe medication, suitable for use by young children and pregnant women. Its main side effect is drowsiness. Another effective antihistamine for acute allergic reactions is hydroxyzine (Atarax®) which is available by prescription. It also has drowsiness as its main side effect. It is a good idea to have the syrup formulations of either Benadryl® or Atarax® on hand because these are more rapid-acting than tablets which need to be digested before entering the bloodstream.

The newer nonsedating antihistamines, such as loratidine (Claritin®), fexofenadine (Allegra®), and cetirizine (Zyrtec®) are also effective, but the tablet formations may not have as rapid an onset of action so they may not be as useful in an acute, potentially severe reaction. They are probably of more use for preventive therapy of hay fever or chronic hives when a daily maintenance antihistamine is required.

When wheezing occurs as a result of bronchospasm and narrowing of the airways in the lungs, inhaled medications called bronchodilators can be used to reverse this narrowing and restore normal breathing. These inhaled medications are part of the standard therapy for asthmatic patients. However, if you have food allergies but not asthma, inhalers might not necessarily be prescribed, unless you have a history of wheezing. Asthma inhalers, especially over-the-counter inhalers such as Primatene Mist®, are inappropriate in the treatment of anaphylaxis and should not be used to treat anaphylaxis without also using epinephrine.

Epinephrine, given by injection, is the drug of choice for anaphylaxis that is life-threatening. Epinephrine is chemically the same as the hormone that our adrenal glands produce in response to stress. It increases heart rate and blood pressure and, in general, prepares the body for trouble. In the event of an acute asthma attack caused by a food-allergy reaction, administration of epinephrine will quickly reverse bronchospasm and stop wheezing. Epinephrine will also stop the leakage of fluid from blood vessels and restore normal blood pressure and heart function. These actions occur in seconds and are life-saving. Epinephrine has a short duration of action and will usually wear off in twenty minutes. Therefore, in a severe prolonged episode of anaphylaxis, it might be necessary to repeat the epinephrine injection. Obviously, the use of epinephrine should be followed by immediate transport to the nearest medical facility for continuation of definitive treatment, monitoring, and follow-up. Epinephrine acts to stimulate the cardiovascular system causing the common side effects of this drug which are increased heart rate, increased blood pressure, and tremor of the muscles. In the situation involving anaphylaxis, an immediate health threat, it is always better to use epinephrine early, and to later deal with any side effects from the epinephrine which are usually transient.

Special Caution for People on Beta Blockers

✦ Beta blockers are a class of drugs used commonly in the treatment of hypertension, migraine headaches, and glaucoma. They are also used in the follow-up care of heart attack patients. Unfortunately, beta blockers block the beneficial actions of epinephrine on heart and lung tissue, thus rendering it ineffective in the treatment of anaphylaxis. Therefore, if you are taking a beta blocker such as Inderal®, Timolol®, Timoptic®, or Lopressor® for hypertension, heart disease, glaucoma, or migraine headaches, consult your physician for appropriate alternate medicines.

Epinephrine is available as an autoinjector for children who weigh less than thirty-five pounds (Epipen Jr.®) and for older children and adults (Epipen®). The Epipen Jr.® contains half the dose of the adult Epipen® and its needle is shorter. The Epipen® is designed so simply that the patient does not need to measure doses or even to see the needle of the injector.

How to use your Epipen®

Remove the gray safety cap. Hold the Epipen® with the black tip against the fleshy outer portion of the thigh. Do not cover the end of the Epipen® with your thumb! Apply moderate pressure and hold for 10 seconds. Pushing the Epipen® against the thigh releases a spring-activated plunger, pushing the concealed needle into the muscle and discharging a dose of epinephrine. You can use the Epipen® directly through clothing. Upon removing the Epipen® after injection, you will see a short needle protruding. The beneficial effects of the drug will be felt within seconds. The most common side-effects are a temporarily more rapid heartbeat and slight nervousness.

The Epipen® delivers only a single dose so multiple Epipens® have to be available if more than one dose is needed. Since epinephrine has a fifteen to twenty minute duration of action, prolonged, severe episodes of anaphylaxis may require repeat doses. Injectable epinephrine is also available as a preloaded calibrated syringe (Ana-kit® and Ana-Guard®). Ana-kit® and Ana-Guard® contain two doses of epinephrine. Smaller doses can be administered by using the 0.1-ml calibrations on the syringe. The Epipen® is the easier device to use and is more widely prescribed and used.

These devices are easy to use and a school-age child can be taught how to use them with minimal effort. The Epipen®, in particular, looks like a large fountain pen and fits in a shirt pocket. No needle is visible even after the cap has been removed, minimizing fear and resistance to self-injection. The epinephrine devices need to be with you at all times, particularly when unanticipated allergen exposure is likely such as when eating outside your home or in school. It is important not to store the Epipen® in the car because epinephrine is not stable in the extreme heat or cold. Most elementary schools require the epinephrine to be kept in the nurse's office so there must be a good plan for the student to have immediate access to the medicine when the nurse is unavailable. Some schools allow the epinephrine to be handed off from teacher to teacher as the students change classes. Most high schools allow for students to carry their epinephrine and self-administer medication with authorization from a physician. Find out if your local ambulance service and the EMTs in your state carry epinephrine. Many states do not allow EMTs to carry epinephrine so you have to be sure you are ready with yours!

Twenty-five to forty percent of people undergoing acute allergic reactions experience **biphasic anaphylaxis** in which the initial symptoms are followed by a delayed wave of symptoms one to four hours later. These symptoms are usually in the form of hives, swelling, and possibly wheezing. The mechanism of biphasic anaphylaxis may be continued absorbtion of allergen from the GI tract and/or the formation and release of additional chemical mediators. The biphasic reaction does not respond to antihistamines. Steroid medications are prescribed to prevent biphasic anaphylaxis, but unfortunately they may not be effective. Because the occurrence of biphasic anaphylaxis is unpredictable, and because medications may not be able to prevent it, I recommend that if you experience anaphylaxis, use your epinephrine and then seek immediate medical attention.

In summary, if you were to ever experience anaphylaxis, the symptoms would be explosive and rapid; evolving in a matter of seconds. The only drug that will work quickly enough to reverse this and save your life is epinephrine by injection. It is the only drug that can simultaneously reverse airway narrowing, tissue swelling, and cardiovascular shock. Antihistamines work much more slowly and have no life-saving properties, but they do effectively reduce the discomfort of itching and hives. Antihistamines *never replace* the use of epinephrine in acute anaphylaxis. Steroids are prescribed to prevent the development of biphasic reactions which can occur hours after the initial reaction but, because they are not always effective, it is best to be observed in a medical facility for at least four to six hours. In the treatment of anaphylaxis, it is better to err on the side of giving epinephrine than not giving it. All physicians are well qualified in the diagnosis and management of anaphylaxis so if you ever have a severe reaction, use your epinephrine and then go to the nearest emergency facility for treatment. *Early recognition and early treatment are the key to the successful management of anaphylaxis.*

WHAT IS THE SMALLEST AMOUNT OF PEANUT THAT CAN CAUSE AN ALLERGIC REACTION?

Daniel was only three-months-old when his parents realized that he was allergic to peanuts. He was still exclusively breast fed and had never been exposed to peanuts before. His father had been cracking and eating shelled peanuts while watching television. When Daniel cried, he picked him up to hold him. Afterward, he was surprised to see a swollen, red, hive-like imprint of his hand on Daniel's back where he had held him.

In most peanut allergy studies, the lowest doses of peanut provoking reactions were in the range of fifty to 100 milligrams (mg) administered in capsule form. To give you an idea of how small a weight this is, one ounce weighs approximately thirty grams, and one mg is 1/1000 of a gram. An average peanut weighs approximately 500 to 800 mg, or one-half to three-quarters of a gram. This means that one-fifth to one-tenth of a peanut can cause a reaction. Hourihane addressed this issue of how small a dose of peanut people will react to in a study published in 1997. He and his colleagues in Southampton, England challenged fourteen peanut-allergic patients with doses of peanut ranging from ten micrograms (ug) to fifty mg. Remember, one microgram is one-thousandth of a milligram, or one-millionth of a gram! The peanut was administered in the form of peanut flour in gelatin capsules. Six of these patients had reacted to crude peanut oil, indicating a very high degree of sensitivity. Only nine reacted to fifty mg, the highest dose in the study. No patient reacted to ten to fifty ug of peanut protein. The lowest dose causing any allergic symptoms was 100 ug in two patients who had mild subjective oral symptoms. The lowest dose of peanut protein causing observable allergic symptoms was two mg, a quantity easily reached by inhaling peanut dust. Two mg is approximately 1/250th of an average peanut.

That microgram amounts of protein can induce allergic symptoms suggests that the potential for contamination is quite high and that quality controls in the food processing, packaging, and manufacturing industry as well as restaurants and food preparation establishments, need to be reexamined. Peanut-allergic consumers of these goods and services need to always be wary of and vigilant about the potential for "hidden allergens" occurring in these tiny amounts in processed foods and eating establishments. This may well apply to other highly allergenic food proteins as well such as tree nuts, fish, and shellfish.

CAN THE ODOR OF PEANUTS CAUSE AN ALLERGIC REACTION?

Elisa, age seven, had only mild asthma symptoms, usually sports-related. She was allergic to peanuts but knew to stay away from them. Riding home from school one afternoon, she was seated next to her best friend who had unwrapped the peanut butter and jelly sandwich she hadn't had time to eat in school. Elisa didn't think anything of it but by the time she got home fifteen minutes later, she was having an asthma attack and needed to use her inhaler.

There are reports in the medical literature of people experiencing allergic reactions merely from smelling the odor of foods they are allergic to. Cooking fumes, in particular, have been cited as triggers of asthma attacks and runny-nose symptoms. The odors of fish and shrimp have been cited as triggers for occupational asthma in workers in the seafood industry. The odor of eggs has also been reported to cause allergic reactions. These allergic reactions are caused by aerosolized food particles generated by cooking and food processing. Other airborne food particles causing reactions have included string beans, lentils, and meats. Dr. John Carlston, an allergist from Eastern Virginia Medical School, reported in 1988 on a 28-year-old woman who had sneezing and itching reactions to the odor of peanut and peanut butter since childhood. The allergy worsened with age and reached a point where nasal symptoms occurred when peanuts were opened on another floor at the far end of the building from where she was located. Subsequently, she developed severe nasal symptoms and an asthma attack while on an airplane after peanuts were served on the flight. There are other similar anecdotal reports of allergic reactions to the smell of peanuts or peanut butter in the medical literature. In 1996, Dawe and Ferguson reported on four patients from the United Kingdom with anaphylaxis to "airborne peanut vapor." The assumption is that there may be sufficient allergenic protein in aerosolized peanut particles to cause an allergic reaction. The minimum amount of protein necessary to stimulate a nerve ending to produce the sensation of a smell is on the order of molecules; a single mast cell can be triggered by one or more molecules of antigen. The minimum number of mast cells required for the development of clinical symptoms is unknown. It has been shown that allergic reactions can be triggered by exposure to microgram amounts of protein. This would be at least an order of magnitude greater than molecular amounts. This phenomenon has not been studied in a systematic manner. There have not been any challenge studies done in a placebo-controlled manner, most likely due to the difficulty of recruiting patients because of the risk of anaphylaxis. Due to the lack of scientific studies, whether or not the odor of a food can cause an allergic reaction remains controversial. Hourihane, from the United Kingdom, believes that many reactions to the odor of peanut are "a psychological aversion and a method of self-defense against true allergic contact [rather] than allergic reactions actually mediated by small volatile proteins." He does, however, state that it is not proven that "extremely sensitive patients would not react to the smell of peanuts and this problem needs to be taken seriously especially in enclosed spaces and those such as airplanes that recycle air supply."

The Medical Board of the Food Allergy Network does not believe that the odor of peanut products would cause a true allergic reaction although it could clearly cause a panic reaction. (Personal communication from Anne Muñoz-Furlong, Food Allergy Network.)

In general, there are four levels of risk involving exposure to food, according to Dr. Robert Wood, director of the Pediatric Allergy Clinic at Johns Hopkins University Hospital. The greatest risk occurs during exposure to foods being cooked. The closer you are to the cooking, the greater the risk. The second level of risk occurs with the manipulation or disturbance of food such as when peanut shells are crushed or swept. The third level of risk occurs with exposure to peanuts in a closed environment with recycled air such as on an airplane. While reactions do occur in this setting and have been reported in the medical literature, as mentioned above, it is still considered a rare problem for most people. The lowest level of risk occurs in the setting where food is being eaten but not cooked, such as in a dining hall or cafeteria, unless there is direct contact with the food.

You need to consider the exact conditions of your environment and your level of exposure and contact to determine your level of risk. How these conditions are modified will usually result from a negotiated compromise, balancing your needs and the similar needs of other allergic people with the needs of the general public. The social and legal ramifications of potential situations in which the public needs conflict with the needs of the allergic individual have not yet been fully played out. These issues will be addressed more fully in a later chapter.

CHAPTER 4

FINDING THE HIDDEN PEANUT PRODUCTS

HOW CAN PEANUTS AND PEANUT PRODUCTS BE "HIDDEN" IN FOODS?

Katherine, age eighteen, was a nationally ranked squash player at Brown University. She was also very allergic to peanuts. After defeating the Wellesley College squash team, she and her teammates went out to a popular restaurant near the campus to celebrate. She ordered chili but did not inquire about nuts because she did not think chili would contain any nut or peanut products. After taking a few mouthfuls of the chili, she felt ill but was conscious and breathing. Her coach drove her to the home of a nearby local physician. He found her in shock. He injected her with epinephrine and called for an ambulance which took her to the local hospital emergency department, arriving at 9:30 p.m. Efforts to resuscitate her failed, and she was pronounced dead at 10:55 p.m. The cause of the anaphylactic reaction was peanut butter used to thicken the chili.

Manufacturers are required to list ingredients on labels, especially highly allergenic foods such as peanut. Careful reading of labels is obviously helpful and important but sometimes not enough. In the

United Kingdom and Europe, peanut can be referred to as "ground-nut," and peanut oil can be referred to as "arachis oil."

The following terms on a package label may indicate the presence of peanut:

Artificial nuts

Beer nuts

Cold pressed, expelled, or expressed peanut oil

Goober peas (slang)

Ground nuts

Imitation nuts

Marzipan

Mixed nuts

Nougat

Peanut

Peanut butter

Peanut flour

The presence of tree nuts may be indicated by the following terms:

Almonds

Almond extract

Artificial nuts

Brazil nuts

Cashews

Chestnuts

Filberts/hazelnuts

Gianduja (a mixture of chocolate cream and mixed nuts)

Hickory nuts

Imitation nuts

Indian nuts (pine nuts)

Macadamia nuts

Marzipan/almond paste

Mashuga nuts (pecans)

Nougat

Nut butters (such as cashew butter)

Nut meal

Nut oil

Nut paste (such as almond paste)

Pecans

Pine nuts (piñon, pignoli)

Pistachios

Walnuts

Adapted from Munoz-Furlong (ed.) *How to Read a Label©*. The Food Allergy Network, 1998. *Used with permission, The Food Allergy Network, 10400 Eaton Place, Fairfax, VA 22030.*

What to Watch Out For

Peanut butter is a popular additive in cooking. Cooks favor its versatility in cooking because it adds extra flavor and texture to many dishes. Peanut butter is often used as a shortening or oil in recipes for many gravies. It can give a smoother texture to sauces and gravies. It is used as a thickener for many recipes. Peanut butter has adhesive properties that allow it to be used to "glue down" the ends of egg rolls to keep them from coming apart. Peanuts, peanut oil and peanut butter are commonly used in many types of international cuisines, particularly Asian cooking. Thai, Vietnamese, Chinese, Japanese, Indian, and Ethiopian cooking are just some of the international cuisines in which peanut and peanut products play an important part. Peanut butter is often used as a flavor enhancer in many Chinese restaurants. Sauces and toppings can have finely crushed peanuts mixed in without any visible sign of them. Peanut sauce is often included as a hidden ingredient in chicken marinade. Peanut powder is a listed ingredient in some vegetable soup mixes. One brand of gourmet popcorn has peanut flavoring to enhance its special flavor. Peanut flour is used in certain brands of frozen dinners. "Slivered almonds" found on some baked goods may actually be made from raw peanuts because they are much cheaper. Peanuts can be reflavored and pressed into other shapes such as those of walnuts and almonds.

Crushed and finely ground peanut shells can be part of the stuffing material of bean bags, "draft blocker bags" that go under doors to prevent drafts, and similar items. Leakage or breakage of these items would lead to aerosol emission of highly allergenic peanut shell particles into the environment. One of my patients had a systemic reaction, with hives and runny nose, on exposure to a bird feeder. The ingredient label listed "peanut hearts." Some arts and crafts projects in schools use peanut butter as an ingredient. Read the labels on store bought arts and crafts projects carefully. Make your child's teacher aware that arts and crafts can be a hidden source of peanut exposure.

The Importance of Cross-Contamination

Cross-contamination of food preparation equipment, utensils, and cookware is an important problem. Because of the demands of practicality in a busy restaurant kitchen, cookware and equipment is reused multiple times for many different entrées. Very small amounts of food that may not be obvious or visible to the cook, particularly oils and liquids, may be left behind to contaminate the next entrée. Studies show that for most food allergies, as little as fifty to 100 mg of food protein can be enough to cause an allergic reaction. However, because the peanut allergen is so potent, even 100 µg of peanut protein (one thousand times less) can induce allergic symptoms in patients. Commercial food-manufacturing equipment can be a source of contamination. The production of nut butters, such as peanut and cashew butters, are often run on shared equipment. The nut and plain versions of many products are often processed on shared equipment. Fortunately, the food industry is now, for the most part, attuned to the reality of food-allergic consumers. It is usually standard procedure for equipment to be thoroughly cleaned between the production of different products, and many companies keep equipment exposed to peanut products separate from other pieces of equipment. Every once in a while you will hear of a company recall of a product contaminated by shared equipment in processing or packaging. Consumers should keep abreast of news reports and alerts from the food industry concerning product recalls and warnings. An excellent source of this information is the Food Allergy Network, which publishes a newsletter and is also on-line (see Appendix A).

Processing Additives

The term "hydrolyzed vegetable protein" used to be commonly found on ingredient labels. Fortunately, manufacturers now are required to list the source of the vegetable protein, so the up-to-date labeling should read "hydrolyzed soy protein" or "hydrolyzed corn protein," etc. A peanut-protein hydrolysate has been used as a foaming agent in soft drinks and as a whipping agent in confections. Hydrolyzed peanut protein is not commonly used in the United States because it is more expensive to produce than corn, soy, or wheat derivatives. However, in other parts of the world, peanut processing is less expensive, so hydrolyzed peanut protein may be more common in food manufactured overseas. Another problem with foods manufactured abroad is that labeling requirements are often inconsistent and less rigorous than in the United States. It would be prudent to avoid hydrolyzed vegetable protein when traveling abroad or when buying international foods which have become available in many supermarkets.

✦ Below is a list of some foods that peanut-allergic people should be cautious of. You need to find out as much as you can about the ingredient list of these foods because they might very well contain hidden peanut products. This is not an all-inclusive list and you need to always read the labels of *all* foods.

Baked goods	Margarine
Baking mixes	Marzipan
Battered foods	Milk formula
Biscuits	Pastry
Breakfast cereals	Nut butters
Candy, especially M&Ms®	Potato Chips
Cereal-based products	Satay dishes and sauces
Chili	Soups and soup mixes
Chinese food	Sweets
Cookies	Thai food
Egg rolls	Vegetable fat and oil
Ice cream	Vietnamese food

Ingredients such as Oriental sauce, emulsifier, and "flavoring" may also contain peanut products. The possibility of cross-reaction with the legume lupine found in flour was discussed earlier. In general, be careful of processed foods as they have a greater potential for containing undisclosed or hidden ingredients including peanut products. Always read labels! I generally recommend limiting your intake of processed foods and eating only those with which you are very familiar. Learning to cook your own recipes with fresh and all natural ingredients is not only allergy safe, but healthier as well.

Intimidating though the above information may be, once you know what to look for and become familiar with certain brand names and ingredient lists, grocery shopping should be easier and more routine. But, don't forget to read those labels because food manufacturing and production methods do change! If you frequent a certain market, befriend the manager and have him special order items for you. If you frequent certain restaurants, let them become familiar with you and your dietary needs. Reward these establishments with your business. Once you establish a plan and routine, eating in or out should remain a pleasurable and safe experience.

WHY AREN'T LABELS FOOLPROOF?

Joshua was diagnosed with milk protein allergy at age three months. He had severe eczema, hives, vomiting, and diarrhea with cow's milk formula and dairy products such as cheese, ice cream, and yogurt. His mother found that a number of food items she bought at the supermarket that were marked "dairy-free" and "Pareve" (Kosher designation for milk-free) caused allergic reactions. These included bakery goods, bread, and non-dairy ice cream.

Labels obviously have to be read and manufacturers are legally required to follow specific guidelines. The Two Percent Rule of The Code of Federal Regulations requires manufacturers to list ingredients that constitute less than two percent of the total weight, but they do not have to be listed in the order by weight. Ingredients in flavors or spices are not required to be labeled nor are incidental additives if they are not functional and in insignificant amount (generally parts per million.) An ingredient can also be listed as a "natural flavoring" to indicate a small amount of a food protein added for flavoring without identifying the actual protein. An example of this is casein (a milk protein) added to canned tuna. There is an excellent article on this subject in the *Food Allergy News*, Aug.–Sept. 1996 issue by Anne Muñoz-Furlong. On some occasions, a manufacturer will change ingredients without changing the labeling. Labels can also be very misleading. For example, "non dairy" products can contain milk protein; "egg substitutes" are low in cholesterol but contain mostly egg white, which is the allergenic portion of egg; and Lactaid® or lactose-free milk lacks sugar but has the same amount of milk protein. It is still most important to know all the possible "code words" listed previously for peanuts, nuts, and allergenic foods that can make reading labels confusing. When in doubt, consult your allergist, the Food Allergy Network, or even call or e-mail the manufacturer.

IS PEANUT OIL SAFE FOR PEANUT-ALLERGIC INDIVIDUALS?

Jane's favorite restaurants were Chinese, Thai, and Vietnamese so when she was diagnosed with peanut allergy, she was crestfallen because she knew peanuts were a staple of Asian cooking. However, she discussed her problem with the managers of her favorite Asian restaurants and they assured her that no peanuts would be used in cooking her meals. Unfortunately, she subsequently had anaphylaxis while eating a seafood dish at the Vietnamese restaurant. The entree contained no peanuts or nuts of any kind, but one of the ingredients had been panfried in peanut oil before being added to the main dish.

Whether peanut oil is safe depends on how it is extracted. Peanut oil is extracted from peanuts by one of two methods. The chemical extraction method extracts the oil by using chemicals, such as hexane, and high-temperature distillation at temperatures of 300°F. or higher. The expeller extraction method makes use of purely mechanical means, with an expeller device, at temperatures from 150 to 200°F. This method has been referred to as "cold-pressed" because of the lower temperatures used as compared to the chemical extraction method. Gourmet cooking oils often are extracted by this method because the oil is more flavorful and is considered more desirable because no chemicals are used. Once the oil is extracted, it can be further refined and purified by several processes that remove free fatty acids, soaps, peroxides, and other impurities that might affect flavor, appearance, or shelf life of the oil.

Several recent studies have analyzed the protein content of peanut oil extracted and purified through these methods. All studies show that chemically extracted and refined oils have negligible protein content and are not associated with reactions when consumed by peanut-allergic individuals. In contrast, the "cold-pressed" or expeller-extracted oils contain peanut protein and can lead to allergic reactions. In general, the oils containing the highest protein concentrations, and hence, the highest allergen levels, are the oils with lowest levels of refinement.

Hourihane studied sixty peanut-allergic patients, challenging them with crude peanut oil and refined peanut oil. None of the sixty patients reacted to the refined peanut oil, whereas six (ten percent) reacted to the crude oil. Another study showed that two brands of crude peanut oil contained ten µg of allergenic protein per milliliter (ml) of oil. Refined peanut oil, on the other hand, had three to five µg of protein per milliliter.

Another problem with cooking oils, particularly in a busy restaurant kitchen, is the risk of cross-contamination of frying different foods in a shared deep fat fryer. In addition, it is common practice for the same frying pan to be used for multiple entrées with the pan being wiped off between entrées. Oil that has been used to cook any peanut product should be considered contaminated with peanut protein.

Because of the significant variability of factory procedures, labeling ambiguities, and inconsistencies, you cannot assume that peanut oil is safe. As mentioned earlier, in manufacturing, peanuts and tree nuts are often processed on the same production lines, resulting in cross-contamination of the final product. Because of these many possible problems, and the severity of the risk involved, I advise peanut- and tree-nut-allergic patients to avoid all nut oils.

CHAPTER 5

KEEPING SAFE IN A PEANUT-FILLED WORLD

SHOULD PEANUT SNACKS BE BANNED FROM AIRLINES?

Elaine is a 34-year-old woman who has had a lifelong history of peanut allergy. Despite always asking about the presence of peanuts in each entrée, she has had anaphylaxis when eating in restaurants on four occasions, and has used her Epipen® each time, effectively treating each episode. On a recent flight to Florida, she experienced sneezing, runny nose, and chest tightness when peanuts were served to the passengers seated in her row. She took Benadryl® which was sufficient to relieve her reaction and did not need her Epipen®. She was moved to another part of the airplane and arrived safely at her destination with no further peanut exposures and no further reactions.

Peanuts have been served on airline flights since the 1950s. As the number of peanut-allergic passengers increased and reports of allergic reactions to peanuts on airlines occurred, complaints to the Department of Transportation prompted an inquiry into this matter. In 1996, an abstract from the Mayo Clinic was published that found peanut allergens could be washed from airplane ventilation filters after 5,000 hours of flight time. Consideration of this study, as well as the Air Carriers Access Act of 1986 which guaranteed access to airlines for the disabled, prompted the department to issue a recommendation in August of 1998, that all airlines provide, on request, a three-row peanut-free buffer zone for a passenger with a medically documented peanut allergy. This resulted in a huge outcry from peanut farmers and the politicians from the peanut-growing states as well as many members of the public offended by a small vocal minority dictating policy. A number of airlines subsequently announced peanut-free flights for peanut-allergic passengers on their request. Policies are subject to change so it is always wise to contact your airline before making reservations.

Airline	Regularly Served Peanuts?	Nonpeanut Snack or Peanut Buffer Zone Available?
American	No (on most domestic flights)	Yes, with a doctor's note
America West	Yes	Yes
Continental	Yes	Not offered
Delta	Yes (regular flights) No (Delta Express, Shuttle)	Yes Not needed
Northwest	Yes	Yes
Southwest	Yes	Yes
U.S. Airways	Yes	Yes
United	No	Yes Not needed

Adapted from Furlong, T.J. "Flying with Food Allergies—Are Airlines Getting It?" *Food Allergy News* Jan. 2000©. *Used with permission from the Food Allergy Network, 10400 Eaton Place, Fairfax, VA 22030-2208.*

The debate that followed resulted in a reversal of this directive. The main objections were: (1) it was an excessive regulation on airlines and ignored the rights of the vast majority of air travelers who are not peanut allergic; (2) the directive unfairly singled out one allergen while ignoring other potentially important allergens; (3) establishing peanut-free zones would establish a precedent for all forms of public transportation. Legislation was subsequently passed that prohibited funding for the Department of Transportation to implement its peanut-free zone directive but encouraged a scientific study of this problem. The lack of scientific studies demonstrating that airborne peanut allergen caused peanut-allergic airline passengers to have allergic reactions was cited as one of the main reasons for not mandating such a strict recommendation.

Researchers at the Jaffe Food Allergy Institute in New York surveyed passenger reports of allergic reactions to peanuts on airlines and published their results in 1999. Sixty-two of 3,704 (1.65 percent) participants in the National Registry of Peanut and Tree Nut Allergy indicated that they or their children had had an allergic reaction to peanut while on a commercial airline flight. Forty-two respondents, with an average age of two years (range of age six months to fifty years), had an allergic reaction that began on an airplane. Thirty-five of the forty-two reacted to peanuts and seven to tree nuts, although three of these could have reacted to something that also contained peanuts. Twenty individuals reacted by ingestion, eight by skin contact, and fourteen by inhalation. The reactions usually occurred within ten minutes, and the severity of the reaction was worse for ingestion followed by inhalation, while the least severe reaction was by skin contact. During inhalation reactions, more than twenty-five other passengers were estimated to be eating peanuts at the time of reaction. Inhalation reactions usually consisted of upper airway symptoms, skin rash, or wheezing. The researchers felt that eleven of the fourteen inhalation reactions were very convincing for true allergic reactions, considering the timing and pattern of the reaction as well as the symptoms experienced. None of these inhalation reactions were life-threatening.

The people notified the flight crews only thiry-three percent of the time. Nineteen subjects received medical treatment in-flight, including epinephrine given to five, and an additional fourteen received treatment on arrival at the gate, including epinephrine given to one and intravenous medication to two.

Airlines have had epinephrine as part of their in-flight medical kits, as required by the Federal Aviation Agency, since 1986. It has been suggested to the airline industry that flight attendants be trained in the recognition of anaphylaxis and the use of epinephrine. Flight attendants should also be notified of passengers with life-threatening food allergies. Passengers should be warned that the airlines make no exceptional cleaning methods for flights. However, the airline might make allowances for allergic people to preboard so they can wipe down their immediate seating area. Passengers should be given the option of allergen-free meals or, ideally, peanut-free flights, if requested in advance. Passengers might be permitted, and encouraged, to bring their own meals if they so choose. This would safeguard them from the possibility of cross-contamination with other meals. None of these suggestions are policy yet, but lobbying and a strong group effort by enough people could certainly result in changes.

Ultimately, even banning peanuts and peanut products from all airline flights would not guarantee safety for the peanut-allergic patient at risk for anaphylaxis. Passengers, particularly children, often bring their own snacks and candies with them and exposure and contact could easily result. There is certainly no way for airlines to prevent this from happening. The false sense of security such flights might engender on the part of both the allergic passenger and the flight crew could end up causing more harm than good. The patient has to take the ultimate responsibility for being vigilant and prepared. The strategy of education and prevention is key. Patients, families, and their physicians can help airlines and their staff understand about peanut allergy; how to recognize and deal with the problems of contact and contamination as well as the handling of an emergency allergy situation. There is no substitute for prudent measures of prevention in dealing with this problem. Families need to always take the initiative and call ahead to inquire about the availability of peanut-free flights. It is a good idea to book the first flight of the day in the early morning to improve the chances of flying on a freshly cleaned and vacuumed airplane. Ask for permission to preboard or board early to clean and wipe down the seating area. You or your child need to bring your emergency medications such as an Epipen®, a bottle of liquid Benadryl®, and any other medications needed (asthma medications, eczema creams, etc.) in a carry-on bag for possible use during the flight. Remember, not only can checked luggage get lost, but it would be useless if an allergic reaction occurred during the flight. Bring your own peanut-free food and snacks so that you or your child don't get hungry and start being tempted by the peanut snacks and other foods of unknown composition. To keep the child from being bored and wanting to explore and wander all over the plane, bring enough toys, games, and other diversions.

WHAT ARE SOME OF THE PROBLEMS FACING THE PEANUT-ALLERGIC INFANT AND TODDLER?

Matthew is a two-year-old boy, who first developed peanut allergy at age one year. He was exclusively breast-fed until age twelve months and was not completely weaned until age eighteen months. He had developed eczema on his face, arms, and legs at two months. The eczema seemed to flare after his mother ate peanut butter and then nursed him. On his first contact with peanut butter, when he touched some on a cracker, he developed swelling of his face, followed by hives all over his body and required Benadryl® and epinephrine in his pediatrician's office. He has been kept on a strict peanut- and nut-free diet since then, and his mother eliminated peanut products from her diet. He had no problems until he was kissed by a relative who had just eaten a piece of candy containing peanut, and hives erupted where he was kissed.

Infants and toddlers are completely under the control of their parents and caretakers. They are a captive audience because they have no control over their environment. How often they get into trouble is directly related to how carefully they are watched and cared for. A strict peanut-free diet and environment can be achieved for this age group more successfully than for any other age group. The ideal situation would be a baby that is exclusively breast-fed by a mother who is herself adhering to a peanut-free diet in a household with no peanut products. Daycare would be avoided completely or at least delayed until age three. Unfortunately, this ideal situation is seldom achieved and is a bit unrealistic. Siblings who are not old enough to understand that peanut butter can be dangerous should not be given peanut products except under supervision so that accidental contacts with and exposure of the allergic child do not occur. The major mistakes occur when care of the child is given over to people who may not be as knowledgeable about peanut-free diets, or who do not care to be. This is where you need to educate others about the seriousness of the allergy and how often peanut products can be "hidden." Any caretaker responsible for the baby needs to be fully trained in handling an emergency situation and in the use of epinephrine. In the daycare setting with multiple children, it is the responsibility of the daycare provider to maintain a safe environment for all her charges. How this is achieved certainly will vary from provider to provider. With very young active children, playing with and touching each other, it is quite difficult to monitor every child. The chances for accidental contact and exposure increase with the number of children present. In an ideal world, the easiest way to maintain control would be to have a completely peanut-free environment.

Since this is often difficult to achieve, it is up to you, as parents, to be in frequent contact with the daycare providers, to give them information, hands-on help, and support.

When looking at various daycare centers, inquire whether they have had children with allergic conditions, such as peanut allergy, and how this was handled. The more experience the daycare provider has had, the more confident you can be about the safety of your child. The Allergy and Asthma Foundation of America (AAFA) has a new program training childcare centers on dealing with food allergies, asthma, and other common allergy problems. Your local AAFA chapter will also direct you to the nearest support group and educational lectures given by community physicians and local experts. This provides an invaluable source of information and a forum for sharing experiences and giving mutual support.

SHOULD PEANUTS BE BANNED FROM SCHOOLS?

Mark, age five, is severely allergic to peanuts and has already had three episodes of anaphylaxis in which one required hospitalization. He has been kept out of preschool because the family could not find a school that satisfied their stringent requirements. They are now about to enroll Mark in kindergarten and are requesting a letter of medical necessity from me and the pediatrician to order that his school prohibit peanuts and peanut products from Mark's classroom as well as from the school cafeteria.

The social and legal aspects of this question are very similar to those related to airline peanut exposure. Some preschools and schools have, in fact, banned peanuts from the classrooms and cafeterias. This has depended in large part on the number of students affected in the school and community, the efforts of the parents to be heard, and the willingness of the school system and community to make accommodations. In most cases, compromise solutions are reached such as having a peanut-free table in the cafeteria or a peanut-free room. This approach is generally quite satisfactory because the actual risk in a dining hall with good ventilation and no exposure to the actual cooking fumes is very low, particularly for anaphylaxis. Students are given age-appropriate education in allergy and what the consequences of anaphylaxis are. The dangers of sharing foods and snacks must be discussed. Hand washing before and after eating greatly decreases the cross-contamination problem. The nurse can use a special light which shows the spots children have missed after hand washing. This helps not only the issue of food allergies, but reinforces good hygiene as well. This education often must begin with the school nurse explaining these issues to administrative staff.

The key to the success of any preventive plan is access to and the availability of epinephrine. This can never be overstated. Without easy access to epinephrine in areas where food and eating occur, potential disaster awaits. This can be a problem, particularly for children who, because of their age, do not have permission to carry their epinephrine with them and are therefore dependent on the school nurse for their epinephrine. Many schools have to share one nurse so an individual school may only have the nurse there a few days of the week. In this not uncommon situation, the nurse has the ability and legal authority in many states to train a designee in the use and administration of the epinephrine. This designee can be a teacher, principal, secretary, or any individual in the school able and available to perform this crucial function in the absence of the school nurse. You need to know exactly what the school nurse's weekly schedule is and to whom she has designated the responsibility for administering epinephrine on the days she is not present in the school. You should have this plan in writing from the school nurse and principal.

Another issue is the school bus and whether the bus driver will have the responsibility for keeping the epinephrine and administering it in an emergency situation. This is a potentially serious gap in your child's preventive plan especially since the school bus is relatively unsupervised with respect to sharing food, snacks, and packed lunches from home. Be sure to raise this issue with the school because they do have responsibility for this part of the student's day as well.

Food Allergy and the Law

✦ It is interesting to note that there have been cases of daycare centers and preschools denying admission to food-allergic children or refusing to allow the administration of epinephrine. *Food Allergy News* has followed the issue of food allergies and the apparent violation of the Americans with Disabilities Act (ADA). There is ongoing litigation involving a number of these cases. The ADA does require the daycare centers to "reasonably modify their policies, practices, or procedures when the modifications are necessary to afford goods, services, facilities, privileges, advantages, or accommodations to individuals with disabilities. That is, unless the public accommodation can demonstrate that making the modification would fundamentally alter the nature of the goods, services, facilities, privileges, advantages, or accommodations." The Supreme Court recently ruled that the ADA does not cover individuals with disabilities that can be corrected or reversed with medical treatment. They felt the intent of the ADA was not to cover "common, correctable impairments and that the person must be limited presently, not potentially or hypothetically." Food-allergic individuals were not specifically dealt with in this ruling, but clearly food anaphylaxis is neither "common" nor "correctable." How the food-allergic patient and the schools are affected will become clearer as legal precedents are set with the cases currently pending in the courts.

WHAT IS THE RESPONSIBILITY OF THE SCHOOL TO THE PEANUT-ALLERGIC CHILD?

A federal law, Section 504 of The Rehabilitation Act of 1973, states that schools must provide medical attention to children who need it, and that budgetary cutbacks are not an acceptable excuse not to do so. The school has responsibility for the child's medical needs during the entire time the student is in attendance at school. State and federal law require that parents provide the school with written documentation of the child's allergies and the physician's signed treatment plan and procedure to follow in the event of a reaction.

The school nurse, or her designee in her absence, will implement the medical plan. The plan should be very specific and list the signs and symptoms to look for during an allergic reaction. Based on recognition of these signs and symptoms, the nurse or her designee will be able to give treatment and medication.

Medication policies vary from school to school. Some schools restrict all medications to the nurse's office. Obviously, this could be a potential problem if the nurse's office is situated a long distance from the eating areas. Death from anaphylaxis can potentially occur minutes after exposure. Ideally the cafeteria monitors will be equipped with epinephrine if this is the case. Other schools have the students' medications in a fanny pack that is handed off from one teacher to the next as the student changes classes. Most schools allow students to carry their epinephrine and asthma inhalers after age ten to twelve, with the written permission of their physician.

It is important for families to provide a **written action plan** to the school and school nurse. Your physician should review the plan. This should be a one-page sheet with the following information: **Student's name** and **personal information** (age, class, address, home and emergency phone numbers, parents' names and emergency phone numbers, and closest relatives or designees from the family to act in the parents' absence)

Physician's name and **phone number.**

Medical information: specific diagnoses

specific allergies

all medications

Signs and symptoms of an allergic reaction:

Skin: itching, flushing, hives, swelling

Mouth: itching and swelling of the lips, tongue, mouth

Throat: itching, swelling, tightness of throat, difficulty swallowing, difficulty speaking, hoarseness, cough

Chest: cough, chest pain or tightness, shortness of breath, wheezing

Heart: weak, thready pulse, dizziness, passing out

Abdomen: nausea, vomiting, diarrhea, abdominal pain and cramps

Action Plan:

1. If peanut product is ingested and only skin symptoms are observed, give (*antihistamine, dose*).
2. If systemic symptoms or anaphylaxis occurs, give Epipen®/Epipen Jr.®/Anakit®. If epinephrine is used, call an ambulance or 911.
3. Call emergency contacts (Mother/Father/Designee)
4. Call physician
5. Call ambulance if emergency contacts or physician are not reachable.

This action plan can be modified for the individual student according to his or her specific history and needs. It needs to be revised as the medical history changes and should be updated at least at the beginning of each new academic year. A copy of this action plan should be kept with the epinephrine. FAN's Emergency Health Care Plan is a convenient form that is reproduced here that you can use as a template for your child's written action plan.

EMERGENCY HEALTH CARE PLAN

ALLERGY TO: _____

Student's
Name _____ D.O.B. _____ Teacher _____

Asthmatic: Yes* ____ No ____ *High risk for severe reaction

Place Child's Picture Here

SIGNS OF AN ALLERGIC REACTION INCLUDE:

Systems	Symptoms:
MOUTH	itching & swelling of the lips, tongue, or mouth
THROAT*	itching and/or a sense of tightness in the throat, hoarsness, and hacking cough
SKIN	hives, itchy rash, and/or swelling about the face or extremities
GUT	Nauseau, abdominal cramps, vomiting and/or diarrhea
LUNG*	shortness of breath, repetitive coughing, and/or wheezing
HEART*	"thready" pulse, "passing out"

The severity of symptoms can quickly change. * All above symptoms can potentially progress to a life-threatening situation!

ACTION:

1. If ingestion is suspected, give_____
medication/dose/route

 and_____immediately.

2. CALL RESCUE SQUAD: _____

3. CALL: Mother _____Father _____or emergency contacts

4. CALL: Dr. _____at_____

DO NOT HESITATE TO ADMINISTER MEDICATION OR CALL RESCUE SQUAD EVEN IF PARENTS OR DOCTOR CANNOT BE REACHED!

Parent Signature	Date	Doctor's Signature	Date
EMERGENCY CONTACTS		TRAINED STAFF MEMBERS	

1. _____   1. _____ room _____
 Relation: _____ Phone _____

2. _____   2. _____ room _____
 Relation: _____ Phone _____

3. _____   3. _____ room _____
 Relation: _____ Phone _____

For children with multiple food allergies, use one form for each food.

Reprinted with the permission of The Food Allergy Network, 10400 Eaton Place, Fairfax, VA 22030.

Personalize Your Child's Items

Pasting the child's photograph on the Action Plan sheet as well as on the child's EpiPen® prescription box for the school nurse makes for easy and quick identification in an emergency situation. Another good idea is to have the younger child eat on a placemat that has his name, photograph, and diagnosis "peanut allergy" on it to further minimize the possibility of mistakes. Printing companies can make stickers on which you can print your child's name, picture, and "peanut allergy." These stickers can be very useful in labeling medications, lunch and goodie bags, placemats, and other items.

WHAT CAN PARENTS DO FOR THE SCHOOL?

Michael's mother became very involved with the school as a result of her son's peanut allergy. She started by talking to his class and answering questions about peanut allergy and how it affected Michael. She then talked to parents about peanut allergy at PTO meetings. She joined the local chapter of AAFA (Allergy and Asthma Foundation of America) and attended their meetings. She subsequently organized lectures and speakers and arranged special programs for the students and parents of Michael's school.

The most important part of any plan is communication and education, and here is where the family has a responsibility to the school. Entering kindergarten and first grade are big landmarks in your child's life. This is the ideal time to establish the educational messages that you as parents will ultimately be responsible for. Most problems that you and your child will encounter result from ignorance. Before school begins, meet with the principal and your child's teacher to discuss your child's specific needs as well as your suggestions for educating the class about peanut allergy. Find out if the school has had students with similar allergic conditions and whether or not they have had experience dealing with medical emergencies. You and your child can do an informal presentation to the class. Contact the Food Allergy Network (FAN) about their School Food Allergy Program. It provides an in-depth discussion for parents and school staff with a food awareness plan. There is also an excellent videotape available from FAN (see Appendix A) called "Alexander, The Elephant Who Couldn't Eat Peanuts" aimed at elementary school children. You can also offer to educate school staff, teachers, and other personnel with

Questions You Need to Ask the School

+ Does the school have a full-time nurse? If not, what days is she there, and who has the responsibility for administering medical care in her absence?
+ Is the student allowed to carry the epinephrine and/or inhaler?
+ What plan do you have in place in the event of a medical emergency?
+ How many peanut- or food-allergic students have you had experience with? Are there any currently enrolled?
+ Has the school ever dealt with an anaphylactic reaction? What was the outcome?
+ What is the closest hospital that a sick student would be transported to?
+ Is the cafeteria peanut-free? Would you provide a peanut-free zone?
+ If my child is the victim of a bully or harassment, how would you deal with that problem?
+ Can we as parents set up an educational forum or discussion group to help educate students, teacher, and staff about peanut allergy?

an in-service presentation. Invite the other parents also. Consider inviting your pediatrician or allergist to be a part of this. I have gone to schools to speak with school nurses, teachers, and students about allergies. Often, the child's physician might be able to provide the in-service teaching as well. I have done this on a number of occasions and find it very useful not only for educating my patients and their families and the school staff, but also for helping my management by improving communication, especially with the school nurse. The school nurse can be the "eyes and ears" for the physician and can be one of his or her most useful allies in caring for patients.

HOW WILL THIS ALLERGY AFFECT MY CHILD'S EMOTIONAL AND SOCIAL DEVELOPMENT?

Michael, aged seven, has had a lifelong history of peanut allergy as well as allergies to tree nuts, dairy products, and eggs. At age five, he had a severe anaphylactic reaction at a birthday party, most likely to nuts. He eats school lunch in a special room separate from the main cafeteria that is "allergy-free." He also has asthma which requires him to use multiple medications during school hours. He dislikes gym and has refrained from participating in team sports. He is constantly teased by classmates and is called "Peter Pan" and the "peanut man." Michael's parents are concerned that he is withdrawing and is depressed and they are consulting a psychologist to counsel him.

One of the more difficult challenges of having a child with a serious and potentially fatal medical problem is the general lack of knowledge that he or she will encounter in the other students and their families. Most people don't understand how dangerous food allergies can be. They also tend to be unaware of the concepts of hidden allergens, cross-contamination, and the fact that very small amounts of an allergenic food can do as much harm as the amount normally eaten at a meal. People feel imposed upon when they have to make personal concessions to situations they do not fully comprehend. They may feel that you are "overprotective" when you ask that peanuts be removed from your child's environment. Therefore, education of the child's classmates and their families is just as important as the education of the school and its staff. This can be accomplished in many ways, both in the classroom and outside school. Meeting face to face with people is generally the most effective way of achieving cooperation. You can arrange to be on the agenda for the next PTO meeting, or invite parents to the classroom setting, or meet in the school cafeteria where some of these potential problems can be made more obvious.

Besides lack of knowledge and ignorance, the other common problem many children face is that of teasing and harassment. Being "different" is likely to make youngsters the target of harassment by other children and food allergy can easily make your child the prey of a bully. Unfortunately, there have been many instances of peanut-allergic children not only being teased but also being physically threatened by other children. There was an example of a bully thrusting an open jar of peanut butter in the face of someone with peanut allergy. The life-threatening potential of this situation makes it more serious than just dealing with another bully, and the consequences are more much more severe than just hurt feelings. This behavior must be dealt with in a swift, definitive way, directly with the school principal. Again, a face-to-face meeting with the offending child's family might be the way to stop this behavior. Many children are unable to comprehend death and life-threatening scenarios may be too abstract for them to understand so they don't realize the consequences of their actions and behavior.

Another consequence of having a serious and potentially fatal medical problem, such as peanut allergy, is in the fear and anxiety that it generates. Particularly in children, phobias toward eating can result especially if the child has experienced a severe allergic reaction already.

It is important that the child understand that, while being careful is good, once safe foods are identified, they can be eaten without fear. Most fears in an older child can be overcome with patience, understanding, and reasoning. In young children, fear can be overcome with support and with the child knowing that there is always someone there to help if he or she gets sick. The child's teacher, school nurse, and principal can be your surrogates during school hours. Familiarizing these persons not only with your child's medical needs but also with his or her specific fears will give your child confidence in them and ultimately enable the child to develop self-confidence.

Because some schools have their food-allergic students sit at special "allergy- or peanut-free tables," these children are separated from their friends and often feel isolated and even punished. Friendships and relationships often suffer as a result. However, many loyal friends will bring peanut-free lunches so they can sit at the table. Again, appropriate education of all involved is the most effective way to prevent problems.

Children often use their medical problems as an attention-getting device, and food allergies are no exception. They may claim that they are experiencing active symptoms such as "trouble breathing," "throat closing," "chest pain or tightness," abdominal pain and "uncontrollable itching," caused by their allergies. It is important to address these symptoms early on and recognize whether they are truly allergic reactions or not. You have to be certain that there was actual peanut exposure associated with these symptoms. Physical signs of an allergic reaction, when present, are important in documenting a true allergic reaction. The presence of redness, rash, hives, and swelling can be helpful. Substantiate symptoms that involve breathing difficulties and asthma with a measurement of lung function with a peak flow meter. You must bear in mind, however, that anaphylaxis need not always present with these symptoms so the severity and urgency of each episode needs to be carefully evaluated by someone with expertise such as the school nurse. If the attention-getting symptoms are rewarded with attention, your child may develop a behavior pattern that will make it very difficult to evaluate future reactions that are genuinely a result of peanut exposure. Professional counseling should be considered if your child's food allergy problem is complicated by this issue.

WHAT ARE SOME OF THE PROBLEMS UNIQUE TO THE PEANUT-ALLERGIC ADOLESCENT?

Jennifer, aged sixteen, has had peanut allergy since age four and has not had any problems with restricting peanut and peanut products. She had a recent allergic reaction when her new boyfriend kissed her after eating peanut butter candy and she developed facial hives. She is very upset today because her boyfriend doesn't seem to understand the seriousness of her allergy and has announced that he shouldn't have to "put up with this" and is breaking up with her. She "wishes she would die and be over with this."

In addition to all of the previously discussed issues, the adolescent presents a unique set of problems. We're all too familiar with the mood swings and occasional rebellious "acting out" behavior of teenagers. All adolescents seek some measure of control and a feeling that they can be independent. Many adolescents express this by deliberate actions to test the limits that have previously been set for them. For the food-allergic adolescent, this may sometimes take the form of either denial or rejection of their allergic condition and ignoring the restrictions placed on them. Such seemingly self-destructive behavior in adolescents is a common problem observed for the entire range of medical problems from diabetes to asthma to smoking, drug and alcohol abuse. A helpful approach might be to involve, for support, friends and peers who might share similar medical problems as well as the adolescent's personal physician or anyone else he or she trusts and respects. Giving the adolescents as much responsibility and control of their lives as possible will reinforce the feeling of trust and confidence they need as they reach for adulthood.

For the at-risk adolescent who already has a tendency towards eating disorders, being on a restricted diet and avoiding food for medical reasons may worsen this problem. Again, early recognition of these issues and early counseling will help prevent the escalation of these problems. Blatantly self-destructive behavior or evidence of eating disorders clearly warrants consultation with a professional counselor.

Just as adolescence is the time to prepare socially, emotionally, physically, and intellectually for eventual adulthood, it is also the time for food-allergic adolescents to prepare to be on their own and to be able to deal with their allergies independently. Certainly, high school is the time to begin this preparation by giving them gradual control. By the time your adolescent is ready to go off to live alone, he or she should be ready for independent living. When looking at colleges in the junior and senior years of high school, visit campuses and inquire about the food services as well as the health services and infirmary. Once the college has been selected, consult the local allergist so that he or she knows your child in the event of a problem. Meet the medical staff and show them your emergency action plan. Forward your child's medical records, especially those of your allergist.

SHOULD YOU WEAR A MEDIC-ALERT® BRACELET?

The Medic-Alert® bracelet is a metal tag engraved with an individual's name and vital information in case of emergency, usually the diagnosis/allergies and brief instructions. The tag can be worn as a bracelet around the wrist or on a chain around the neck. Its purpose is to provide life-saving information in case the patient is unable to give it because of either age or incapacity. In addition, the responding person can call the Medic Alert's twenty-four Hour Emergency Response Center which has a computerized data file on the person with medical history and other vital information. Obviously, in the event of loss of consciousness due to an anaphylactic reaction, a passerby can be immediately informed of the patient's diagnosis by reading the Medic-Alert® bracelet and, if so instructed, administer life-saving epinephrine. Whether or not a peanut-allergic patient chooses to wear the Medic-Alert® bracelet depends on the risk of fatal anaphylaxis and the risk of the patient being incapacitated to the point where he or she is incapable of self-administering the epinephrine or communicating with other people. The use of the Medic-Alert® bracelet in very young children would be for the remote possibility of their being left alone without adult supervision. A young child should always be under the supervision of a responsible adult well-versed in the child's specific allergic condition and the management of an allergic reaction, including the use of epinephrine. Of greater concern is the young child who is not quite old enough to understand and articulate the specific problem, but is just old enough so that he or she might not always be under constant adult supervision. This is the child at the greatest risk for an accidental ingestion, often resulting from sharing and playing with other children. This age group is usually the late preschool to early elementary school grade level. Generally, older children and adults do not have any of these issues and the main reason for wearing the Medic-Alert® bracelet would be in case of encountering the situation where loss of consciousness or incapacity occurs. The wearing of the bracelet can sometimes interfere with sports or get caught on playground equipment, so this needs to be looked out for. The Medic-Alert® bracelet comes in several sizes and styles and can be fairly unobtrusive. You can obtain ordering information from your doctor or contact Medic-Alert directly by calling (800) 432-5378 or writing to 2323 Colorado Avenue, Turlock, CA 95382.

CHAPTER 6

PREVENTION OF PEANUT AND OTHER FOOD ALLERGIES

SHOULD YOU AVOID PEANUTS AND OTHER ALLERGENIC FOODS DURING PREGNANCY?

Jill had a craving for peanut butter during her first pregnancy and admitted that every chance she had, she ate peanut butter sandwiches, peanut butter spread on crackers, cookies and fruit. Her love for peanut butter continued through the three-month period she nursed her baby. Gregory, now two, developed peanut-allergy symptoms the very first time he was exposed, with hives on his mouth and face. Jill just found out that she is pregnant again and wants to know if she should eliminate peanut products from her diet.

There is evidence that the fetus has the capability of making immune responses and, specifically, it can make IgE responses to milk and egg proteins as well as to some environmental allergens. There are two studies that examine the effect of avoiding allergenic foods during pregnancy on the development of food allergies and allergic disease in infancy. Maternal avoidance and elimination diets did not prevent the development of allergic diseases, including food allergy in either study.

In spite of these findings however, the British Medical Council has recommended the avoidance of peanuts and peanut products by all pregnant and nursing women with newborns at high risk for allergies. These potentially allergic babies would have either personal or family histories of allergies, asthma, or eczema. This recommendation may have been influenced by Hourihane's 1997 study, showing that there is a relationship between increased maternal consumption of peanuts during pregnancy and lactation and earlier onset of peanut allergy in infancy and childhood. The increasing numbers of peanut- allergic individuals as well as the permanence of peanut allergy are also factors to consider in making this recommendation. Although there are no guarantees, giving up peanuts during the time of pregnancy and breast-feading could potentially prevent your child from experiencing this life-threatening allergy.

IS BREAST-FEEDING HELPFUL IN PREVENTING FOOD ALLERGIES?

Ellen's first baby was bottle fed with infant formula. He was colicky in the first two weeks and needed several formula changes until things got better with a soy formula. At age two months, he developed eczema at about the same time foods were added to his diet. He was diagnosed with milk, egg, and peanut allergy by the pediatrician with positive RAST tests at age six months. He wheezed for the first time at age ten months when he had viral bronchitis. Since that time, he has wheezed with colds and respiratory infections. He is now three and wheezes with active play and running. His pediatrician feels that he has asthma. Ellen is pregnant with her second child and asks if breast feeding this baby will help prevent what her son had to go through.

Breast-feeding in the first year of life is recommended by most pediatricians and by the American Academy of Pediatrics. Human breast milk is nutritionally complete and contains everything the newborn and infant need to grow and develop. Breast milk also contains numerous components of the immune system that help the baby defend against infection. These include protective antibodies which increase natural immunity, and various enzymes that can kill bacteria, in addition to other protective elements of the immune system. Because of these benefits, all babies should be nursed, regardless of their risk for allergic disease.

Since allergic diseases which include not only food allergy, but allergic rhinitis (hay fever), asthma, and eczema are all genetic and inherited, the baby who has relatives with these allergic diseases is at a greater risk for developing allergic diseases. If one of your parents has allergies, your chances of developing allergies is about thirty-three percent. If both of your parents have allergies, your chances of developing allergies is about sixty-six percent. But remember, these are just statistical probabilities of the potential risk of allergies. You can help determine what actually happens to your child in real life by nursing exclusively and following specific strategies.

The importance of breast milk with regard to allergies is that it is nutritionally complete so no other foods need to be given with it. The exclusively breast-fed infant does not need to be exposed to numerous "foreign" proteins that may be sensitizing. If the nursing mother is able to avoid eating allergenic foods such as peanuts, tree nuts, and shellfish, the baby's exposure to sensitizing proteins is even less. For a discussion on eating peanuts while nursing, please see page 25. The newborn and infant gastrointestinal tract is a very complex system which must be capable of breaking down and absorbing foreign nutrient proteins, while at the same time rejecting and fighting foreign bacterial and viral proteins that are harmful to the body. If, because of immaturity, the baby's GI tract is ineffective in modifying and processing the allergenic aspects of these food proteins, inflammatory and allergic reactions to these proteins can result, causing the baby to become sensitized. By breast feeding exclusively in this critical first six months, when the gut is most immature, exposure to foreign proteins and allergens is significantly reduced and the likelihood of developing allergies is lessened. No one knows exactly at what age the gastrointestinal tract has matured enough to be able to adequately process and handle foreign proteins without significant risk of sensitization. In general, many experts feel that by age three years, the child's GI tract is able to handle most allergenic foods and is therefore at a reduced risk for developing food allergies. For this reason, many experts now recommend that the child with the most risk factors for being allergic to foods (having a personal history and/or family history of allergies, asthma, and eczema), be restricted from the highly allergenic foods, such as peanuts, tree nuts, and shellfish, until the age of three years.

WHAT IS A REASONABLE SCHEDULE FOR THE INTRODUCTION OF FOODS INTO THE DIET OF A POTENTIALLY FOOD-ALLERGIC INFANT?

There are no universal recommendations or policies with regard to this question. Based on available information from studies, most allergists would recommend strict breast feeding for at least four to six months. There is some controversy in regard to this, but I would recommend the mother restrict highly allergenic foods from her diet, including peanuts, tree nuts, and shellfish, to minimize the risk of sensitization through breast milk. Nursing supplements or weaning can be done with an elemental or hypoallergenic formula such as Neocate®, Elecare® Nutramigen®, Pregestimil®, or Alimentum®. These products are available in most pharmacies and many supermarkets. Solids should be delayed until age six months and begun with the least allergenic foods first such as rice cereal, fruits, and vegetables. Individual foods should be added sequentially weekly or biweekly, one food at a time. Animal proteins, which are more allergenic, should come after the fruits and vegetables which tend to be less allergenic. Hold off on cow's milk and eggs until age twelve months. Highly allergenic foods, such as peanut, tree nuts and shellfish, should ideally be held off until age three years. Some conservative recommendations would hold off on the introduction of peanuts and nuts until age five years.

Age to Introduce Food	Food
Birth to 4–6 months	Breast milk
4–6 months	Rice cereal, fruits, and vegetables
6–12 months	Wheat, oat, cereal grains, dairy, soy, egg, chicken, turkey, beef, lamb, pork Introduce individual foods sequentially, one food per week.
12 months	Fish
36 months–5 years	Peanut, tree nuts, shellfish

CHAPTER 7

THE FUTURE OF PEANUT ALLERGY

CAN PEANUT ALLERGY BE TREATED WITH ALLERGY SHOTS?

Allergy shots, or allergen immunotherapy, has been in use for the treatment of hay fever and asthma since the early 1900s. This form of treatment works by inducing an immunity to the various environmental allergens, such as pollens; molds; dust mites; and animals, by regular monthly injections of the allergenic material in graded minute amounts over a period of three to five years. Since the 1970s, allergen immunotherapy has been successfully used in the treatment of insect-sting anaphylaxis from honeybees, yellow jackets, hornets, and wasps by the administration of minute amounts of insect venom over five years or more. For patients meeting the selection criteria, the success rate of immunotherapy for hay fever is as high as eighty percent, with the possibility of long-term remission of symptoms. The success rate for venom immunotherapy is even higher, at ninety to ninety-five percent, effectively curing this potentially fatal allergy. Usually, the main side effects of immunotherapy are allergic reactions localized to the site of the injection, but occasionally systemic reactions do occur.

Immunotherapy For Food Allergy

The use of immunotherapy for food allergy was first reported by Freeman in 1930. He was able to desensitize a seven-year-old boy who had unstable asthma triggered by fish ingestion, as well as hives, angioedema (swelling), vomiting, and diarrhea with fish exposure. The patient lost both his fish allergic reactions and his skin test reactivity to fish. He was able to maintain his desensitized condition by eating fish and taking cod liver oil every day. There were almost no subsequent reports of treatment of food allergy with immunotherapy in the subsequent decades because the standard treatment for food allergy continues to be avoidance and an elimination diet. In 1987, Dr. John Carlston, of Eastern Virginia Medical School, published on the successful treatment of two patients with food allergies with food immunotherapy. The first patient had peanut allergy with anaphylaxis, including allergic symptoms caused by inhalation of peanut odor. She was treated with injections of peanut extract, starting at a dose of 0.05 ml of a 1:100,000 weight per volume dose that was gradually increased 150-fold to a maintenance dose of 0.5 ml of a 1:2,000 dose. This maintenance dose is the equivalent of 1/10th of a teaspoon of a solution made by mixing one gram of peanut in two liters (more than 2 quarts) of water. This is a minuscule amount of peanut! She had frequent allergic reactions to treatment including wheezing, but she did lose her peanut sensitivity. After a year of symptomless peanut exposures, her immunotherapy was stopped. She continued to do well on follow-up one year later. The second patient reported was a seafood restaurant worker whose asthma was exclusively triggered by her working environment. She was treated with a mixture of fish (cod, flounder, halibut, mackerel, and tuna) and shellfish mix (clam, crab, scallop, oyster, and shrimp). Her asthma improved greatly, allowing her to work without symptoms, and she was also able to eat shrimp without problem.

In 1992, Drs. Nelson and Leung and their colleagues at the National Jewish Medical and Research Center in Denver,

Colorado published a randomized placebo-controlled study of peanut immunotherapy in patients with a history of peanut allergy and anaphylaxis. Eleven patients began the protocol and eight patients reached maintenance immunotherapy. Of the four patients finishing the study, three received peanut immunotherapy and one received placebo. The three patients who received peanut immunotherapy had a significant decrease in symptoms on DBPCFC and a decrease in skin test reactivity to peanut. The placebo-treated patient had no change in either DBPCFC or skin test reactivity. Unfortunately, systemic reactions occurred at the very high rate of 13.3 percent, almost four times that of pollen immunotherapy. This study is the first to demonstrate, in a well-controlled manner, that traditional immunotherapy can be an effective treatment for food allergy and anaphylaxis, dispelling the old dogma that immunotherapy for food is ineffective.

Presently, immunotherapy for food is still considered experimental because of the high incidence of side effects and the lack of larger, more extensive controlled studies documenting safety of the treatment.

WHAT DOES THE FUTURE HOLD FOR THE TREATMENT OF PEANUT ALLERGY?

There are presently many exciting areas of research in food allergy. Better understanding of the immunology of allergic reactions as well as progress being made in the identification and characterization of peanut allergens with gene sequencing may one day make it possible to manipulate the immune response to these allergens. Once this becomes possible, it might be possible to "turn off" the allergic response.

One approach is to decrease the amount of circulating IgE in the patient. Antibodies to IgE can be made which will bind to and remove IgE from the circulation. Since the presence of IgE is required for all allergic reactions, this theoretically could be the answer to all types of allergic diseases from food allergies to hay fever to eczema to asthma. These anti-IgE antibodies have already been studied in mice with good results, and several human trials in patients with hay fever and asthma show promising early results. Drs. Leung and Nelson at the National Jewish group in Denver, and Dr. Sampson's group in New York have begun a multi-center study, including Boston Children's Hospital and Arkansas Children's Hospital, to examine the effects of anti-IgE injections in the prevention of peanut allergy.

Another novel approach to treatment is a DNA vaccine which contains the DNA coding for peanut allergen Ara h2. Injection of this DNA induces a suppressive immune response that "turns off" the response to Ara h2, thus preventing any allergic reaction to peanut. This approach is being tried in mice and rodent models and hopefully can be applied to humans in the near future.

The main drawback to traditional immunotherapy with peanut extracts is the very high rate of allergic reactions both local and systemic to each injection. There is certainly a risk of anaphylaxis as well, if an incorrect dose or error is made in the administration. To counteract this problem, the immunotherapy material may consist of peanut protein that has been modified to contain only the portion that is recognized by the patient's immune system, but that lacks the portion that will bind to IgE on mast cells. In this fashion, the immune system will be able to generate the same type of immunity to peanut while at the same time, there would be no chance for any allergic reactions to the injections because the allergen would be incapable of binding to mast cells. This type of immunotherapy has been called **peptide therapy** because only the relevant portion of the whole peanut protein, called the peptide, is administered in the injection. Peptide immunotherapy has already been studied in human trials with cat allergen and ragweed pollen allergen, and hopefully peanut peptide immunotherapy will be tested in the future.

Another approach to the problem of food allergy is to make the food itself nonallergenic, or hypoallergenic, through genetic engineering. Characterization of the three peanut allergens Ara h1, Ara h2, and Ara h3 has identified the portions of peanut protein that bind to IgE. It is this binding of the peanut allergens to IgE that triggers the mast cells to release histamine and the other chemical mediators causing allergic symptoms and anaphylaxis. Without binding of IgE to the peanut allergens, no allergic reaction would occur. Since the genetic structure and sequence of the three peanut allergens is known, scientists are now able to alter the peanut protein and render it incapable of binding to IgE. Through genetic engineering, a new type of peanut could be grown containing these altered proteins, and these peanuts would not trigger any allergic reactions in peanut-allergic patients. Genetically engineered plants have already been available for years now with qualities such as resistance to pests and disease, enhanced nutritional content, longer shelf life, and many other desirable features. The technology now exists to greatly reduce the allergenicity of foods and to make foods safe for all to eat.

WHERE CAN I LEARN MORE ABOUT FOOD ALLERGIES?

The best single source of information on food allergies in general is your local allergy specialist. He or she has the special training to help clarify your various symptoms and make the diagnosis of specific allergies. Most importantly, he or she can give specific recommendations on allergy-control measures and avoidance strategies and give you the most current treatment based on the newest advances in allergy and immunology research. He or she will work with your primary care doctor in formulating a well-thought-out and reasonable plan for managing your food allergies.

For the best resource available to the public on food allergies, the Food Allergy Network (FAN) is unparalleled. They are a non-profit organization that serves "to increase public awareness about food allergies and anaphylaxis, to provide education, and to advance research on behalf of all those affected by food allergies." The organization was founded by Anne Muñoz-Furlong whose daughter was diagnosed with milk and egg allergies as an infant. Lack of information and support for people and families with food allergies prompted her to form this organization which is now not only the best resource for patients and families, but is also involved in funding research and educational programs. It is very active in the food and restaurant industry and in government and legislative issues as well. FAN formed the National Registry of Peanut and Tree Nut Allergy for all peanut- and nut-allergic people to register and provide information about their allergy history. This registry provides a valuable database from which a number of important medical studies have already originated.

FAN is on-line at http://www.foodallergy.org. Their address is 10400 Eaton Place, Suite 107, Fairfax, VA 22030-2208 and their telephone number is (800) 929-4040. They publish a bimonthly newsletter for adults and a separate one for children. They have many publications on specific topics, including peanut allergy, tree nut allergy, and understanding food labels. They have a useful cookbook and recipes are included in every newsletter. They have excellent school programs as well as instructional videotapes, including one I highly recommend, "The Elephant Who Couldn't Eat Peanuts." One of the most useful services to patients are "Special Allergy Alert Notices," which keep the public up to date on the food industry's latest news bulletins, recalls, and warnings on products. I recommend FAN to all my patients with food allergies.

Other sources of information on food allergies or allergic diseases in general are the Allergy and Asthma Foundation of America (AAFA); the American Academy of Allergy, Asthma, and Immunology (AAAAI); and the American College of Allergy, Asthma, and Immunology (ACAAI). AAFA provides educational programs to the general public and local support groups for patients and families with asthma and allergic diseases, including food allergies. AAAAI and ACAAI are professional organizations for allergy and asthma specialists, but they do provide information and educational materials to the general public on asthma and all allergic diseases. They also have a referral directory so that patients can be given names of allergy and asthma specialists in their local communities. Both organizations have web sites and can be found at **www.aaaai.org** and **www.acaai.org** respectively.

WHAT ARE THE MAIN TAKE-HOME POINTS TO REMEMBER ABOUT PEANUT ALLERGY?

✦ Peanuts are one of the main causes of food allergies and, together with tree-nut allergies, are the leading cause of fatal and near-fatal food anaphylaxis.

✦ The incidence of peanut allergy has increased by fifty percent over the past 20 years.

✦ Most people do not outgrow peanut allergy (only ten–twenty percent), unlike most other food allergies.

✦ The symptoms of allergic reactions are itching, hives, swelling of face, throat, tongue, abdominal pain, vomiting and diarrhea, difficulty breathing, wheezing, dizziness, loss of consciousness, and shock.

✦ Anaphylaxis is a systemic reaction that can lead to cardiovascular collapse and death. It requires immediate treatment with epinephrine.

✦ Since there is no cure as yet for peanut allergy, strict avoidance is the key to management.

✦ Accidental ingestions are a fact of life. Twenty-five percent of peanut-allergic patients have had accidental ingestions and reactions in the preceding year.

✦ Be prepared to deal with accidental ingestion and anaphylaxis when eating and traveling outside the home. The peanut-allergic individual should have epinephrine on his or her person wherever contact with food is expected, especially outside the home. He or she should also have a rapid-acting liquid antihistamine such as diphenhydramine (Benadryl®) or hydroxyzine (Atarax®).

✦ Epinephrine is the only drug that will treat anaphylaxis. It is better to overtreat with epinephrine rather than undertreat.

✦ You should create a written action plan with your physician and file it with the medical office at the workplace or nurse's office in school.

✦ Learn to read labels and ingredient lists.

✦ Be aware of the problem of hidden allergens, cross-contamination, and indirect exposures.

✦ When eating outside the home, inform people of your allergy; especially food servers, restaurant staff, school cafeteria staff, airline staff, and so forth.

✦ Peanut oil may not be safe if it has been contaminated through cooking or if it is crude, cold pressed, or unrefined.

✦ Peanut allergy is caused by a specific immunologic response to peanut protein.

✦ Peanut allergy is usually genetically determined and inherited.

✦ Peanut allergy is more common in an individual who has other allergic diseases, such as hay fever, asthma, or eczema, and is more common in close relatives such as siblings, parents, and other relatives who have allergic diseases.

✦ Parents with allergic diseases will have children at higher risk of developing allergic disease, including food allergy.

✦ Confirm the allergy with a consultation with an allergist who can evaluate the problem with allergy testing.

✦ The gold standard for the diagnosis of food allergy is the double-blind placebo-controlled food challenge (DBPCFC).

✦ Potentially allergic infants should be breast-fed for the first six months to minimize exposure and sensitization to food proteins. Ideally, the maternal diet should not contain highly allergenic foods such as peanuts, tree nuts, and seafood.

✦ The highly allergenic foods, such as peanuts, tree nuts, and seafood should be withheld from the potentially allergic child's diet until age three years. In general, this appears to be the general age at which the child's immune system and gastrointestinal tract is able to handle and process these highly allergenic foods.

✦ Knowledge of the molecular structure of the peanut allergens may enable the development of novel vaccines to treat peanut allergy. Advanced biotechnological techniques may lead to new strains of genetically engineered peanuts that do not cause allergic reactions.

✦ Until then, education, increasing public awareness, and prevention remain the principal approaches to this increasingly common problem.

GLOSSARY OF TERMS

Allergen A substance that causes an allergy. In the case of food, this is usually a protein.

Allergic Rhinitis An allergic condition characterized by nasal congestion, itching, sneezing, and mucous, usually caused by environmental allergens, and commonly called "hay fever" which is a misnomer because patients don't get fever and the allergen is not hay!

Allergy An abnormally high sensitivity to certain substances such as food, pollen, medications, or bee stings.

Anaphylaxis A severe, generalized, systemic allergic reaction characterized by hives, swelling, difficulty breathing, wheezing, and gastrointestinal symptoms. **Anaphylactic shock** is characterized by a drop in blood pressure in addition to the aforementioned symptoms and is life threatening.

Angioedema Swelling of tissue. When angioedema occurs in a critical area, such as the throat or tongue, obstruction of breathing can result in a life-threatening reaction.

Antibody A protein produced in response to foreign substances such as bacteria, toxins, and **allergens**. Antibodies are essential elements of the immune system in the response to infection as well as allergic reactions. The antibodies that neutralize bacteria and viruses are IgG and IgM. The antibody produced in allergic reactions is **IgE**.

Antihistamine A drug that counteracts the effects of **histamine** by binding to **histamine receptors** on tissues. This makes it important in treating allergies of all types since histamine causes the symptoms of allergic reactions.

Asthma A chronic inflammatory condition of the lungs, resulting in difficulty breathing, cough, chest tightness, and wheezing. It is commonly triggered by infection, allergy, and physical factors such as exercise and cold air temperature.

Atopic dermatitis The medical term for eczema.

B Cell A white blood cell that produces antibodies such as **IgE**.

Biphasic anaphylaxis An anaphylactic reaction in which the immediate symptoms are followed by a second wave of delayed symptoms hours later.

Bronchospasm Spasms of the airways in the lung causing obstruction and resulting in the symptoms of **asthma**.

Casein A white, tasteless, odorless milk protein. It is the basis of cheese and is also used to make adhesives, plastics, and paint.

Conglutin One of the allergenic peanut proteins.

Cross-Reaction The reaction between an allergen and IgE generated against a different but similar allergen, often belonging to the same family or category. For example, a person who is allergic to walnuts and experiences anaphylaxis to pecans has had a cross-reaction between walnuts and pecans.

DBPCFC Double-blind placebo-controlled food challenge; the "gold standard" for diagnosing food allergy. In this procedure, neither the person tested nor the doctor (double blind) will know if the placebo or the actual food is given. This procedure eliminates any bias factor from the study.

DNA The genetic material found in cells that determines individual hereditary characteristics.

Eczema A chronic inflammatory skin condition often associated with allergic triggers such as food or environmental allergens. It is more common in people and their relatives who also have asthma and allergic rhinitis.

Elemental Diet A prepared, nutritionally complete **hypoallergenic** diet consisting of basic nutrients such as amino acids, fatty acids, and simple sugars all of which contain no allergenic proteins. It is in liquid form and available for infants, children, and adults.

Elimination Diet A diet that has strictly and completely eliminated the specific food(s) you are allergic to. Children who adhere to their elimination diet are more likely to outgrow their food allergy.

Epipen® An automatic injector of the drug epinephrine which is the drug of choice for the treatment of anaphylaxis.

Epinephrine The drug of choice for anaphylaxis which relieves the skin, cardiovascular, gastrointestinal, and respiratory symptoms of an acute allergic reaction.

Gene A hereditary unit located on a chromosome that determines specific characteristics of the organism. Genes consist of DNA sequences. See **Gene Cloning** and **Gene Sequencing.**

Gene Cloning The technique of making multiple identical copies of a gene.

Gene Sequencing Determining the order of the unique DNA structure of a gene which can allow **cloning** of the gene, eventually leading to synthesis of the protein.

Gluten The main allergenic protein in wheat.

Glycinin One of the allergenic peanut proteins.

Glycoprotein Any protein containing a carbohydrate sugar component. Most allergenic proteins are glycoproteins.

Histamine A physiologically active chemical released by **mast cells** as part of the allergic reaction. Histamine causes all the symptoms of allergy such as itching, sneezing, swelling, mucous production, and wheezing. The actions of histamine are blocked by **antihistamine** medications.

Hydrolysate The product of hydrolysis, a chemical reaction that breaks down and degrades a chemical or food, such as soy or milk hydrolysate. Hydrolysates are not necessarily less allergenic than the parent compound.

Hypoallergenic Having a decreased potential to cause allergic reactions.

IgE The antibody, produced by B cells, that recognizes allergens. **Mast cells** attached to IgE will bind to specific allergens which will result in the release of **histamine**. The resulting effects of histamine on the body are what we recognize as allergic symptoms.

Immunology The study of the structure and function of the immune system.

Immunosuppression Suppression of the immune system by drugs, radiation, or by diseases such as malignancies and AIDS. When the immune system is suppressed, it no longer performs many of its functions such as recognizing self from nonself and fighting bacteria and viruses.

Intolerance An adverse reaction to food that is not mediated by the immune system. In gastrointestinal intolerances, it is due to an inability to digest certain foods. For example lactose intolerance.

Lactalbumin One of the **whey** proteins in milk.

Lactoglobulin The other whey milk protein.

Mast Cell One of the key cells of the immune system involved in allergic reactions. Mast cells bind **IgE** and produce and release **histamine**. Mast cells are found in all the target organs of allergic symptoms such as skin; eyes; mucous membranes of the nose, sinuses, ears, lungs; blood vessels, and the gastrointestinal tract.

Mediators Chemicals made by cells of the immune system that *mediate* various reactions in the body such as allergic reactions.

Ovalbumin An egg-white protein.

Ovomucoid Another egg-white protein.

Peptide Therapy A form of allergy therapy that involves injections of only the active allergic component (peptide) of the allergic protein. The theoretical advantage of this form of allergy injection is that there are much fewer allergic reactions and side effects to the injections.

Placebo A substance that contains no active ingredient as does a food or drug. It is used in medical studies as a control for patients who believe they are being given the active ingredient.

RAST RadioAllergoSorbent Test; is a blood test that measures the level of **allergen**-specific **IgE** in your blood to determine if you are allergic to that allergen. It is almost as accurate as a skin test.

Receptor A molecular structure or site on the surface of a cell that is able to bind to chemicals, such as **histamine**, or to proteins, such as antibodies like **IgE**.

Skin Prick Tests Skin tests are performed by pricking a pointed instrument or device through a drop of allergenic extract that has been placed on your skin. The skin is not broken, but the prick enables enough fluid extract to penetrate the first layer of the skin. An allergic skin reaction comparable to a small mosquito bite will form if you are allergic to that allergen. Skin prick tests are a reliable way to diagnose allergies.

Tropomyosin A muscle protein that is the main allergen in shellfish.

Urticaria The medical term for **hives**: a skin rash characterized by very itchy red welts, usually caused by exposure to an allergen.

Vicilin An allergenic peanut protein.

Whey The watery part of milk that separates from the curds (also known as **casein**) when milk curdles. Whey contains **lactalbumin** and **lactoglobulin**.

APPENDIX D

REFERENCES

The references I have cited throughout this book are listed below for the more ambitious of you, who wish to go to the primary sources. In addition to the sources below, *Food Allergy News*, the newsletter of the Food Allergy Network (FAN) is an invaluable reference source. Also available from FAN, is a compilation of all the peanut-allergy articles previously published in that newsletter.

Bernhisel-Broadbent, J. and Sampson, H. "Cross-allergenicity in the legume botanical family in children with food hyper-sensitivity." *J Allergy Clin Immunol* 1989; 83:435–440.

Bock, S.A. et al. "Double-blind, placebo-controlled food challenge (DBPCFC) as an office procedure: A manual." *J Allergy Clin Immunol* 1988; 82:986–997.

Bock, S.A. "The natural history of food sensitivity." *J Allergy Clin Immunol* 1982; 69:173–177.

Bock, S.A. "The natural history of peanut allergy." *J Allergy Clin Immunol* 1989; 83:900–904.

Burks, W., et al. "Peanut allergens." *Allergy* 1998; 53:725-730.

Carlston, J.A. "Injection immunotherapy trial in inhalant food allergy." *Annals Allergy* 1988; 61:80–82.

Dawe, R.S., and Ferguson, J. "Allergy to peanut" (letter). *Lancet* 1996; 348:1552.

De Montis, G., et al. "Sensitization to peanut and vitamin D oily preparations." *Lancet* 1993; 341:1411.

Ewan, P. "Clinical study of peanut and nut allergy in sixty-two consecutive patients: new features and associations." *Brit Med J* 1996; 312:1074–1078.

Ewan, P. "Prevention of peanut allergy." *Lancet* 1998; 352:4–5.

Fries, J. "Peanuts: Allergic and other untoward reactions." *Annal Allergy* 1982; 48:220–226.

Gerrard, J.W. "Allergy in breast-fed babies to ingredients in breast milk." *Annal Allergy* 1997; 100:596–600.

Hourihane, J. "Peanut allergy—current status and future challenges." *Clin Experimental Allergy* 1997; 27:1240–1246.

Hourihane, J. "Peanut allergy: recent advances and unresolved issues." *J Royal Society Med* 1997; 30 (suppl):40–44.

Hourihane, J., et al. "An evaluation of the sensitivity of subjects with peanut allergy to very low doses of peanut protein: A randomized, double-blind placebo-controlled food challenge study." *J Allergy Clin Immunol* 1997; 100:596–600.

Hourihane, J., et al. "Peanut allergy in relation to heredity, maternal diet, and other atopic diseases; results of a questionnaire survey, skin prick testing, and food challenges." *Brit Med J* 1996; 313:518–521.

Hourihane, J., et al. "Randomized, double-blind, crossover challenge study of allergenicity of peanut oils in subjects allergic to peanuts." *Brit Med J* 1997; 314:1084–1088.

Hourihane, J., et al. "Resolution of peanut allergy: case-control study." *Brit Med J* 1998; 316:1271–1275.

James, J. "Airline snack foods: Tension in the peanut gallery." *J Allergy Clin Immunol.* 1999; 104:25–27.

Jones, R.T., et al. (abstract). "Recovery of peanut allergens from ventilation filters of commercial airliners." *J Allergy Clin Immunol* 1996; 97:423.

Koerner, C. and Hays, T. "Nutrition basics in food allergy." *Immunol Allergy Clin NA* 1999; 19:583–603.

Legendre, C., et al. "Transfer of symptomatic peanut allergy to the recipient of a combined liver-and-kidney transplant." *N Engl J Med* 1997; 337:822–823.

Lehrer, S. et al. "Immunotherapy for food hypersensitivity." *Immunol Allergy Clin NA* 1999; 19:563–581.

Loza, C. and Brostoff, J. "Peanut allergy." *Clin Exp Allergy* 1995; 25:493–502.

Mulherin, K. "Day care center sued for discriminating against food-allergic children." *Food Allergy News* 1997; 6(3):3.

Muñoz-Furlong, A. "Food labeling rules, practices, and changes to come." *Food Allergy News* 1996; 5:3.

Oppenheimer, J., et al. "Treatment of peanut allergy with rush immunotherapy." *J Allergy Clin Immunol* 1992; 90:256–262.

Plaut, M. "New directions in food allergy research." *J Allergy Clin Immunol* 1997; 100:7–10.

Rix, K., et al. "A psychiatric study of patients with supposed food allergy." *British J Psychiatry* 1984; 145:121–126.

Rosen, J., et al. "Skin testing with natural foods in patients suspected of having food allergies: Is it a necessity?" *J Allergy Clin Immunol* 1994; 93:1068–1070.

Rosen, J. "Treatment of anaphylaxis at home and at school. A guide for physicians." In press.

Sampson, H. "Food allergy. Part 1: Immunopathogenesis and clinical disorders." *J Allergy Clin Immunol* 1999; 103:717–728.

Sampson, H. "Food allergy. Part 2: Diagnosis and management." *J Allergy Clin Immunol* 1999; 103:981–989.

Sampson, H. "Food allergy and the role of immunotherapy." *J Allergy Clin Immunol* 1992; 90:151–152.

Sampson, H., et al. "Fatal and near-fatal anaphylactic reactions to food in children and adolescents." *N Engl J Med* 1992; 327:380–384.

Sampson, H. "Managing peanut allergy." *Brit Med J* 1996; 312:1050–1051.

Sicherer, S., et al. "Clinical features of acute allergic reactions to peanut and tree nuts in children." *Pediatrics* 1998; 102(1). URL:www.pediatrics.org/cgi/content/full/102/1/e6.

Sicherer, S., et al. (abstract). "Peanut allergy in twins." *J Allergy Clin Immunol* 2000; 105:181.

Sicherer, S., et al. "Prevalence of peanut and tree nut allergy in the United States determined by a random digit dial telephone survey." *J Allergy Clin Immunol* 1999; 103:559–562.

Sicherer, S., et al. "Self-reported allergic reactions to peanut on commercial airliners." *J Allergy Clin Immunol* 1999; 103:186–189.

Steinman, H. "'Hidden allergens in foods." *J Allergy Clin Immunol* 1996; 98:241–250.

Teuber, S., et al. "Allergenicity of gourmet nut oils processed by different methods." *J Allergy Clin Immunol* 1997; 99:502–507.

Weeks, R. "Peanut oil in medications." *Lancet* 1996; 348:759–760

Wood, R. "More answers to commonly asked questions about anaphylaxis." *Food Allergy News* 1999; 8:6.

Yuninger, J. "Lethal food allergy in children." *N Engl J Med* 1992; 327:421–422.

Yunginger, J., et al. "Fatal food-induced anaphylaxis." *JAMA* 1988; 260:1450–1452.

Zeiger, R. "Prevention of food allergy in infants and children." *Immunol Allergy Clin NA* 1999; 19:619–646.

Michael C. Young M. D. received his A. B. from Harvard University and graduated from Yale Medical School. He trained in Allergy and Clinical Immunology at Children's Hospital in Boston. He is on the faculty of Harvard Medical School and practices at Children's Hospital, Boston and South Weymouth, Massachusetts. Dr. Young is a past president of the Massachusetts Allergy Society and was recently selected by the Center for the Study of Services for *The Guide To Top Doctors*.